JEAN MARK LABASQUE

COVID-19

THE PROBLEM AND THE SOLUTION

Effective
Countermeasures
for the Great Reset

ISBN: 978-1-66780-625-9

eBook ISBN: 978-1-66780-223-7

NO EVIL SHALL BEFALL ME AND MY FAMILY, NOR SHALL ANY PLAGUES COME NEAR OUR DWELLING.
PSALMS 91:10

TABLE OF CONTENTS

FOREWARD

Sir Isaac Newton is reputed to have said that, "If I have seen further than others, it is because I was standing on the shoulders of giants." No author works in a vacuum and relies on hundreds of previous authors for information and ideas. This work is no exception to the rule. A lengthy bibliography is included to give credit to all. Five authors in particular stand out for their guidance in solving this hoax. Gregory Lessing Garrett's **The Invisible Enemy** and **The Age of Deception** were essential in uncovering the problem. Former New York Times reporter Alex Berenson's **Unreported Truths about Cojvid-19 and Lockdowns** gives all the statistics and references on how the pandemic was misrepresented for political and economic ends. Lt. Lawrence Frego's **An End to All Disease and the DaVinci Code Revelations** provided the solution. Dr. Joseph Mercola and Ronnie Cummins new classic **The Truth About COVID-19: Exposing the Great Reset, Lockdowns, Vaccine Passports, and the New Normal**. Lastly Patricia Cori's **Atlantis Rising, The New Sirian Revelations** and **The Cosmos of the Soul** provided a spiritual perspective of the Secret Government and offered some hope for the future of the Earth and mankind. You will also want to see Mike Adam's Global Reset Survival Guide a free eBook at www.brighteon.com. And no bookshelf would be complete without a copy of the Tools for Freedom catalog. www.toolsforfreedom.com.

The paramount problem for society currently is that an arrogant, dishonest, elite scientific community wants to rule by controlling technology. Make no mistake, this is the ultimate battle between good and evil as predicted in the bible. These unelected and unwanted leaders want to set up a scientific totalitarian and worldwide criminal enterprise. And they want to steal your soul in making everyone a mind-controlled slave. The hope of the wicked is a one world government under Satan and a 90% reduction of the human population. Covid-19 is merely a false flag operation towards this end. As you will learn in this book the devastation caused by lockdowns was unnecessary and could have been prevented for as little as .60 cents per HCQ tablet. The Secret Government powers that be assumed no one would ever crack the Covid-19 hoax. They were wrong!

Jean Mark LaBasque

COVID-19: The Problem and the Solution

By Jean Mark LaBasque

INTRODUCTION

I HAVE BEEN ON THIS planet for 70 years but have never experienced a year like 2020. It appears that the world has indeed gone to hell in a hand basket. There have been riots, murders, looting, hurricanes, forest fires, and worst of all COVID-19. This is World War III for the planet.

Conspiracy theories abound about the creation and dissemination of a virus. First, let me say that the term "conspiracy theories" is a term coined by intelligence agencies to discredit whistle blowers who reveal classified or sensitive information. If the information cannot be discredited, then Option B is to kill the whistle blower and thereby stop the leak of information. More high-profile defectors cannot be killed so they are charged with treason or something convenient and jailed. Then they get killed. That is how the game is played.

Covid-19 is a classic scenario of an intelligence black book job. The red flags start to fly when scientists and doctors go missing and are presumed dead. Dead ambassadors and constant denial are also red flags. Whenever the red flags start to accumulate it is time to investigate what is going on for the safety of the public.

Another word we need to define is "disinformation." This is a Soviet Cold War term meaning lies and propaganda. A couple other classic examples are "green moneys caused HIV" and "Moslem terrorists attacked the World Trade Center on 9/11." Covid-19 is no exception. We know this as Satanists think they are smarter than us and they sign their work. The hidden meaning of Covid-19 is "see sheep surrender." Therefore, we can be assured the virus hoax is a bio-warfare operation of the highest magnitude just like HIV and brought to you by the same lovely folks. Therefore, we need to establish the truth in order to formulate effective countermeasures.

This book is divided into two parts: The Problem and the Solution. The threat is infinitely greater than you can even imagine. Both aspects will take time and effort to unravel the puzzle palace, but complete UNIVERAL IMMUNITY is possible for those who are willing to do the spiritual work needed. Let me say that a spiritual problem (disease) cannot be totally solved by mechanical means alone. If you cannot wait to get started, then just skip to part two and read part one at your convenience and in any order. The whole text of important summaries will be included in the appendix as stand-alone articles and may be reprinted in total. The authors hereby give permission to reprint.

It will be necessary to cover a lot of ground in this volume as getting the big picture will take some background investigation. Evil has been around for millions of years, so it is imperative the reader understands how it operates and why.

If one starts with an open mind and realizes that everything you have learned since birth is a lie, then you will be on the right track.

We will cover everything from the beginning of Earth to the nature of God and Man. We will begin and end with man's true nature as a being of light and love.

You have been TOLD that the only way to prevent a pandemic is to either create herd immunity or use a vaccine. In the absolute best-case scenario these are only effective for a particular disease until such time as a disease mutates. Annual revaccination may be necessary until the disease is either eradicated or becomes so resistant the vaccine treatment is no longer effective. Unfortunately, this is all a lie as the vaccines may kill more people than the disease itself and could lead to altering the DNA of the entire population. The vaccines could lead to mass sterilizations and worse. The entire pandemic may be a hoax and the cures are being withheld for political ends. A glass of concord grape juice daily or dandelion greens may be more effective in preventing the flu that all the vaccines, but THEY don't want you to know that. The fake pandemic may also spell the end of personal liberty and the full exploitation of the police state.

Vaccine manufacturers may have cooked the books to make it appear their vaccines are effective and safe, while they may only be as little as 1% effective. The common cold is a Coronavirus therefore we may have already achieved a herd immunity and all the fear mongering is just a lot of hype. And there will be a certain number of deaths due to allergic reactions in healthy individuals. Those who already have several comorbidities may experience an overreaction called the cytokine storm. Many of these will die also. As the MRNA type experimental vaccines have never been evaluated on animals or humans it is possible there will be mass deaths a couple years down the line as vaccines LOWER immunity. Dr. Judy Mikovits estimates 50 million deaths from the vaccines. I would estimate up to 25% fatalities in certain elderly populations. That is their goal. However, there is another way to long lasting health and protection against all disease.

What you have not been told is that there are ancient ways to create Universal Immunity that have been used effectively for tens of thousands of years. I have named this technique **THE ASCENSION PROTOCOL** and part II of this book explains how to accomplish this holistic protocol to create **Universal Resistance to ALL DISEASES.**

CHAPTER 1

OF GODS AND MEN

THERE MAY BE 100,000 HABITABLE planets in our galaxy alone. It is also likely that over 100 different races of beings exist in this vast space. I would estimate that more than 50 races have visited Earth in the past and that several still reside here in secret. A complete guide to 82 alien species is entitled: The Extraterrestrial Species Almanac: The Ultimate Guide to Greys, Reptilians, Hybrids, and Nordics by Craig Campobasso. Many of them are indistinguishable from us and in fact they are us. However, some look more like Fabio on the good side and the creature from the black lagoon on the far end. I was not too shocked to see the Archangel Michael listed as an alien.

A modern religion, the Baha I Faith teaches about the alien races. Their founder professes that: "Know thou that every fixed star has its own planets, and every planet its own creatures, whose number no man can compute." See The Baha I Faith and Aliens: The Evidence Revealed by Grace J. Keene, JD. They believe in a New Age of peace, prosperity, and possible alien contact.

You may think I am off target beginning this discussion in a book about politics, disease, economics, warfare, and healing, but I assure you it is extremely relevant. Bear with me.

Intelligent beings embodied in the 3rd dimension have been around for millions of years prior to the creation of humanity on planet Earth. Unfortunately, distinct species have been at war with each other for eons and whole planets and civilizations have been destroyed. The same is true for our solar system. Our asteroid belt was formerly a planet called Marduk. It was exploded during interstellar wars.

Earth was a remote waystation during the period of interstellar warfare and was settled by various species of beings, most notably those of the reptilian races. The human races were originally developed as recently as 400,000 years ago. Humanity was created by master geneticists to be perfect vehicles of light with a blend of 5 different species from 5 different planets each. They were designed by enlightened masters to live to over 1,000 years of age and to have full spiritual powers with 24 strand DNA. The different races of humans and blends were created in this way for survival against a harsh environment. Each race was given its own special survival attributes. We are ALL a mixture of all races.

The original inhabitants of Earth were NOT pleased by the encroachment of humans. The reptilian races did everything in their power to destroy humanity, lower their genetic capacity, and shorten their lifespans and enslave them. Humans were first enslaved to mine gold and precious metals in Africa for their masters. This trend continues to the present day.

The enslavement of humanity is where the historical record begins. The Bible records in GENESIS 6:4 that when "the sons of (the) God(s) saw the daughters of men and took them as wives." Thus, began the hybridization of humankind and the mixture of reptilian DNA which is hard wired into our brains. This intermarriage of species did not in any way end the extreme hatred that the reptilian races had for humanity. In fact, it increased it. The reptilian races remain committed to enslaving humanity and contemptuously view us like cattle to be slaughtered and eaten or a sexual plaything. As many as 1 million children are reported missing every year for this reason.

The historical trend of enslavement has existed for millennium. I cannot impress this upon you enough. It is the root cause of all present problems. The only thing that has changed is that enslavement has become more sophisticated. Virtually all aspects of life on this planet are geared to control and enslave the human race. Once you understand this historical background everything in the puzzle palace will start to make sense. It is not just evil, greed or corruption that are behind the forces at play. It is a deeply engrained feud of constant warfare that has existed in the Galaxy for millions of years. It has always been all out warfare. We are the most modern recipients of it.

Humanity advanced technologically over the period of 300,000 years and began to resist the reptilian races or the forces of darkness (the fallen angels of the bible.) Atomic warfare was conducted over the Indus Valley over 40,000 years ago and the valley has traces of radioactivity to this day. The Biblical Sodom and Gomorrah are also radioactive, and the sands of Arabia have extensive areas of molten green glass from atomic detonations. Somehow the pilot's manual from these ancient Vimana aircraft have survived and complete plans are published. Those of you who doubt the existence of the alien presence should read these accounts. And read up on all the pyramids and ancient structures there are around the world that could not possibly have been built by the hand of man.

The ancient continent of Atlantis sank during the incessant warfare due to a massive explosion caused by scaler energy directed through the Earth. This occurred about 12,500 B.C. It is fortunate that the Earth itself was not destroyed. Due to this never-ending warfare the reptilian population has been reduced to just a few thousand. The bad news is that they still control the entire Earth with the help of their countless ruthless minions. Understanding how "the system" of enslavement works is the key to our freedom. This will be the focus of the problems we currently face.

Humanity was not destroyed by the sinking of Atlantis or the Biblical flood. In both instances some people were informed enough to flee before calamity stuck. Survivors flourished at various locations around the Mediterranean and the Middle East. The Pyrenes in Spain and Egypt were popular destinations. Civilization as we know it was rebooted with the introduction of agriculture, animal husbandry, metallurgy, architecture and the building of cities. This was due to alien visitors of the period who set themselves up as Gods and ruled through their vassals who they installed as kings and high priests. Detailed accounts of this rebirth were recorded on clay tablets in cuneiform around 6,000 B.C. Historian Zacharia Sitchin (www. sitchin.com) translated the cuneiform tablets for decades until his death in 2010. He published 10 volumes about life in the Middle East and ancient Babylon under the rule of the Anunnaki Gods. It is fascinating reading and sets the stage for modern times.

The Anunnaki "Gods" had weapon systems and technology 1 million years more advanced than those on Earth as all the advancements of the Atlanteans' were on the bottom of the ocean. I cannot prove that the "Gods" had weapons like Flash Gordon's and Dr. Ming's death Ray, but I think it is highly likely. It is easy to maintain law and order when you can vaporize the dissidents. However, for day to day control of the peasants the "Gods" established kings and their divine right to rule as they acquired their authority directly from "the God" himself. To exercise control over the minds of the people a class of high priests were established and only they had physical access to "God" and everyone else was unworthy. A peasant who unknowingly touched an alien artifact such as the Ark of the Covenant was at once killed by electrocution. This greatly enhanced the power of the "Gods" and their supernatural powers.

There are several Biblical accounts of high priests and prophets meeting with "God" which are clearly alien encounters. The most notable being the meetings of Ezekiel and Moses. The shock and awe presence of the "Gods" appeared to have waned over time. The "Gods" lamented that the people no longer followed the old ways. Many colonizing Gods may have evacuated and returned to their home planet Niburu the 10th planet when it returned on its 3,500-year passage by Earth. Or they may have decided that subsurface secret cities were a safer locale to live away from the huge population of unruly subjects. Regardless, the system of kings and priests was solidly enthroned to rule over their subjects with or without any contact from the Gods above or below.

Kingship eventually evolved into a larger feudal system with kings who rewarded vassals with land, gold, titles and women. These created Lords of the Manor owed allegiance to the king and supplied military service when called upon. The common man had few freedoms as his manorial lord was judge, jury and executioner. The divine right of kings to rule was not significantly challenged until the Magna Charta in 1215. The concepts of free men and common law took a long time to develop under British law and made its way to the American colonies.

The high priest class held great power under "God" and the king. It would be fair to say that the ancient priests of Egypt, Israel, and Babylon were second only to the king. They were well educated and knew the ancient mysteries and the true history of the Earth. They used their knowledge to rule the people and control their beliefs. The priest class amassed great wealth due to their mastery of both alien technology and spiritual practices. They sometimes usurped the power of weaker kings. However not all the practices employed were of the light. Quite the contrary some employed the forces of darkness and what we now term Satanism. Black tantric sexual abuse, torture and murder are how the Global elite gain their power in Satanic rituals.

Now a couple extremely, important points must be made. First, the priest class ALWAYS kept 2 sets of books. One for themselves and one for the masses. To ensure knowledge and power was not leaked to underserving eyes extensive use of codes, codewords, and anagrams were employed. Knowledge is power and it was to be solely confined to the ruling class. For example, the Bible was never intended to be revealed to the common man even though the most secret knowledge was encrypted. The encryptions are numerological, meaning each letter has a number value which relates to a code book. The code can only be decoded in the original language. If a passage or book is translated into another language all you have left is the fake cover story. You have the garment not the body. This information is discussed in more detail in the DaVinci Code Revelations.

Inevitably the question arises about a "sacred" text being "the word of God" or "divinely inspired." Therefore, we must first define God. I define God as the creative force of the universe. This force is the frequency of love. The more you access this force the more blessed and God-like you become. A true spiritual master can be a co-creator with God and materialize objects with mind alone. Remember Jesus turning water into wine as an example. This is something the bad guys of the ruling class do not want you to know as anyone can do it with training. That is why there is a total backout of the truth.

Earlier we talked about colonizing Anunnaki visitors setting them-selves up as Gods with their high technology and possibly spiritual powers as well. They set up rules and religions for the people to maintain law and order. These laws are NOT necessarily divine or universal laws. I would argue that the 10 commandments of Moses are indeed universal law, but every paragraph of every alleged sacred text must be scrutinized to see whether it adheres to the universal law of love of the creator. The mere act of recording an idea or event down does NOT necessarily make it sacred or true. Discretion is always valuable.

Many individuals in this day have great spiritual and psychic powers. This process has remained unchanged since the days of the prophets. The greater one's spiritual calibration and degrees of knowledge the more capable one becomes. A psychic can channel people, spirits, entities, records from anywhere in the universe. This can be an extremely exciting endeavor and extremely rewarding if used in the service of mankind. However, we all must be aware that every entity, spirit, alien, or energy force in the universe is not necessarily benevolent. Quite the contrary. Some spirits and aliens love to play practical jokes on unsuspecting humans who think they are talking to God. Do not be fooled.

The Bible says God's house has many mansions. I believe this refers to the many dimensions of consciousness. We are all living in 3rd dimensional reality AT THE MOMENT. However, there may be 12 levels of consciousness. The higher levels of consciousness DON'T REQUIRE A PHYSICAL BODY. They exist as pure energy with the creator and CAN manifest a body whenever they feel like it. Whether or not a disembodied soul is of the light or chooses the darkness is totally up to them as all souls have free will to choose.

My old friend David Childress used to have a bumper sticker on his refrigerator that read "just because they're dead doesn't mean they're smart." I always got a kick out of that and its good advice. My mother could see and speak to ghosts, but I have only seen one benevolent one. The bottom line is that anyone who receives information from the other side or other dimensions of consciousness is not necessarily receiving God's truth or anything near it. He or She could have a trickster on the party line having fun with you. And God forbid you channel in a malevolent spirit. I have seen 80 of them and they are ugly. Again, every recorded line of spiritual texts MUST be examined for the truth of the laws of love and light. Surround yourself with Gods' golden light daily to protect yourself.

The use of "sacred texts" to keep the unaware under control is as old as our present civilization. Most Christians are not aware that the Bible has been edited 27,000 times. Nor are they aware that the books chosen for the bible were voted on by a council of drunken whoring fist-fighting bishops at the Council of Nicaea (modern Turkey) in the year 325. Reading of the texts not chosen such as the Gospel of Mary Magdalene, can shed a lot of light on what the bad guys do not want you to know. Modern keepers of the status quo have gone to great lengths to keep original tests from public scrutiny. (Such as the Nag Hammurabi texts.) All religions have some truth to them. The challenge is to separate the truth from the lies planted by the forces of darkness to manipulate us. Fake news has been around a long time!! We must all understand that there is a great deal of evil in the world as well as the good and we will explore this. Only by understanding the enemies of truth can we set ourselves free. It only takes the mistranslation of a couple words to totally give the wrong meaning to a passage. For example, our mainstream depiction of Jesus is that of a lowly carpenter. He is allegedly a master crafts-man, which readers of the bible have assumed is a carpenter. However, if we translate this passage as a "master of the craft" then we can see Jesus was an alchemist and holder of the secret knowledge. References to the wives of Jesus and his children have been cut as the bad guys do not want anyone to gain enlightenment by means of tantric sexual yoga from India. This secret is encoded in many forms of Western art as to the sexual prowess of Christ. It appears all the great masters such as Buddha and even the Mohammad were tantric masters.

The false belief that only Jesus can heal is prevalent. The bottom line is that the forces of darkness have conspired to obscure all the paths to enlightenment as they don't want anyone to escape their control by becoming co-creators with God by following the example of Jesus or Buddha. I have channeled Jesus a few times and he is not the man you think he is. He loves to sing and dance and has a profound sense of humor. He is a fun guy!! Do not be misled.

Once interstellar trade is reestablished in the extremely near future a great deal of religious dogma will disappear faster than a kite in a hurricane.

CHAPTER 2

THE MONEY PYRAMID

SEVERAL DECADES AGO, I STARTED practicing a concept called "millionaire's mind." I reasoned that if I diligently studied the actions and methods of "The Rich and Famous" that armed with this knowledge, I eventually would become a millionaire myself. It was a simple but workable concept. So, I read many cases of books, attended 5 colleges, graduated from one, and completed 33 military schools- many at the top-secret level. I studied everyone, networked my way into ultra-prestigious clubs, attended ambassadors' parties, and worked the rooms. Hollywood producers, magnates, and Queens and Presidents have invited me to do lunch. Not bad for an old country boy. Beats milking cows- I can tell you that!!

I really believe in The American Dream painted by Napoleon Hill, Norman Vincent Peale, and others. Emigrants can still pass Lady Liberty and arrive with a suitcase and a dollar and become wealthy and successful in one generation. Those who access The Divine Mind and partner with God always make it eventually. No power on this Earth can keep a good man down or a bad man up.

Our creator has given each of us the power to access either his light or to sink in the quicksand of darkness. Light and darkness are always operating in world consciousness. So, it is a question of choice which power we choose to access and follow. We know a great deal about the Horatio Algers among us, who acquire their wealth, power, and prestige by operating in Divine harmony and work for all to see in the light of day. However, the man in the street, who sleepwalks through life unaware of the forces around him, is almost totally unaware of those who work in secret and in darkness intent upon doing evil deeds. The purpose of this essay today is to shed the light of day upon this darkness. Evil cannot survive in the light of day. It is my duty to inform you, my beloved, of the shape of things to come so they can be prevented.

Every story has a beginning, and every problem has a root cause and effect. On this, the fourth great civilization to inhabit the Earth, the story of good and evil begins in ancient Babylon. As we have previously discussed, this was the period of history when "The Gods of Heaven" saw the daughters of men and took them as wives. The "Gods" of Heaven created the kings of the Earth. Combining their genetic material with that of man, they created Adam and Eve in a test-tube. Almost at once, the new creations divided into two camps. One group was in favor of enlightening humanity and the other wanted them as slaves in the fields and gold mines. Guess who won?

Jesus was a direct genetic link to those who wished to instruct humanity and his seed are very much alive and well today. Even though some have fallen into darkness. The "other' camp came to be known as the Aryan or "Master Race." Master is a key word here as it signifies the desire on their part to enslave all those they feel are below them. Which of course is everyone but himself or herself. Their leader is the "Satanic archetype" commonly referred to as Lucifer. He is their false god. I used the collective word archetype because what we are talking about is a distinct race of beings and not an individual per se. They are physically represented in bodily form on the Earth and inhabit the spiritual realms of the next or fourth dimension.

13

It may immediately come to mind- "How do we distinguish these evil ones from the good ones if they both look just like us?" It is easy. Just as the Bible says, you know them by their works! The Aryan "bad guy" lines are characterized by exceptionally high intelligence, cleverness, greed, deceit, treachery, and unparalleled evil mostly done in secret with their compatriots. In modern psychological terms, we can define these people as megalomaniacs, sociopathic personality types, mass murderers, and totally missing the gene for compassion, pity, love or remorse. Their reptilian brain is dominant. They have no right and wrong. It is all about THEM. In essence, they look human, but they behave more like machines. Think of the character Hannibal Lector in a suit, and you have pretty much got it. They will eat your liver if you are not careful and wash it down with a fine chianti. Or sell your bodily organs while you are still alive to watch. Without the benefit of an anesthetic of course!

About 500 years ago the merchants of Venice, Italy discovered a technique today called fractional reserve banking. This allowed them to create money out of nothing and they financed the Renaissance and the wars of the period. The Aryan bloodlines flocked there in masse, and with their cunning and treachery, they amassed the first great fortunes. The more wars they financed at exorbitant interest, the more money they made. This is an extremely important concept as the tradition continues to this day. Naturally, they financed both sides. With their newfound wealth, they intermarried with European royalty and become known as the Black Nobility. Eventually, the Black Nobility infiltrated almost every royal line with the intent to be the powers behind the thrones and backed it up with their great wealth. One of the Aryan Black Nobility bloodlines went to Germany. Originally known as Baer, they changed their name to Rothschild or Red Sign as this was their coat of arms. The new Rothschilds were goldsmiths, and they created a fractional reserve banking system from the gold that was left in their safe. Eventually, they played their clients' money and amassed a tremendous fortune. Mayer Rothschild sent his 5 sons to five cities to create banks and an empire. These banks evolved into central banks, whereby all the money for the entire country was created out of nothing and used to finance countries' wars, corruptions, mistresses and evil. All the while looking very respectable. The Rothschild creation known as the Bank of England is the most notable. The first bank of the United States was created after the American Revolution, but its charter was cancelled by President Andrew Jackson. After many financial panics created by the Rothschilds, they were able to sneak in the Federal Reserve Bank in 1913- a private Rothschild bank. All our money and gold were then siphoned off to Europe. Long story.

At the top of the money pyramid, we have the 13 Black Nobility families who own most of the world. I call them "the Satanic 13" for simplicity. Others call them the Illuminati, the Power Elite Bankers, banksters, the powers that be, the establishment, the New World Order, the man, the military-industrial complex, the Deep State, the swamp, the Fourth Reich, the Shadow Government, or simply THEM. The Rothschilds alone are believed to own 50% of the Earth, up 25% since WWI and $70 trillion dollars in gold. $500 TRILLION IN ALL.

Next, through a vast, vast system of banks, multi-national corporations, dummy corporations, interlocking directorships, political leaders, intelligence organizations and secret Satanic societies, etc. the Black Nobility runs or controls most of the Earth. In addition to the Rothschilds and their close associates the Warburgs, Schiffs, Prince Bernard, Gettys, Rockefellers, Morgans, Mellons, Vanderbilts, round out the top 10. We really do not know for sure whether these families are the 1st string, i.e., of the Satanic 13 or the 2nd string their underlings. Either way, they are at the tip of the pyramid. The bottom line is that the bad guys control trillions of dollars and use this wealth to promote their agenda of a New World Order under Satan. This is what is happening right now!! A complete list of the players can be found in the book **Blood Lines of the Illuminati by Fritz Springeier.** This edition was published in 1998. The latest editions are in 3 parts and available on Kindle.

Next on the pyramid, we have the United Nations. As some of you are aware, the U.N. was built on the east side of New York City on land bought for

$8.5 million and donated by the Rockefeller family- one of America's premier Satanic Black Nobility families. **The land given to the U.N. was the site of old cattle slaughterhouses and was chosen for its negative vibration. There were so many slaughterhouses on the 16 acres it was nicknamed "Blood Alley." The pure and beautiful land offered on the hills in Philadelphia was rejected because brotherly love was not what the Satanic 13 had in mind.** Scores of millions died in WWI and WWII to create it as a vehicle of control. **Convicted Soviet spy Alger Hiss wrote the UN charter.** As the League of Nations created after WWI was unsuccessful a more devastating war had to be created with WWII to get the U.N. into being. When the New World Order does not get what they want they punish the entire world to get it. Naturally Wall Street and the power elite bankers financed both sides of both wars. The game plan is ALWAYS to create something so horrible that the masses would beg for something to be done. Author David Icke called this the Problem Reaction Solution scenario. This is how the power elite create their wars and how they created all their structures of control. Remember this!! This is what Covid-19 is all about. Control.

The stated purpose of the U.N. is to create peace through a one world government, a one world bank, one world army, one world court, and one world currency. The U.N. did not mention the part about the one world religion. Sounds like Utopia, doesn't it? Well, the devil is in the details. What they did not put into the brochure, of course, is a one world religion dedicated to Lucifer. With a micro chipped population hard wired to the beast. The latter would allow them to control the emotions of the masses. And with tracking software know the location of everyone. Anyone who objects to being a Communist slave gets rounded up and whacked! Cradle to grave control by the brotherhood and they plan to cull the population by 90%. Opps. That was not in the brochure either! We will talk about all this later in the book. There are a lot of logistics involved in killing 7 billion people. But do not worry- they have a plan.

Naturally controlling the ignorant masses and making all their decisions for them is a big job. Next on the pyramid, we have all the 2nd and 3rd

level decision makers united with the formation of various world organizations that support the New World Order objectives of the U.N. Under this category, we have the British Round table, created by imperialist Cecil Rhodes, then, the Bilderberg Group, the Council on Foreign Relations in New York City, the Club of Rome, the World Economic Forum, and many more. The purpose of these organizations is to control the political, diplomatic, economic, military, and intelligence affairs of their respective host countries. And thereby conduct the orders of the Satanic Brotherhood to enslave the rest of the world! The directorships of all these organizations are linked to all the banks and all the other layers in the system- just like a gigantic multi-level chess game.

"Players" is a good description of the world's major political leaders. All are just actors, puppets on a string. Like secret agents for evil, (Manchurian candidates) they are selected, sometimes, if possible, as early as birth from the "bloodlines" and groomed to assume positions of power, leadership and deceit. Bill Clinton, Barak Obama and George Bush are New World Order poster boys. They were often seen making Satanic hand gestures to the unsuspecting. George Bush often praised the New World Order on camera. I suspect that gay Nigerian Communist Barack Obama (aka Barry Soweto) was conceived in a Satanic ritual and if you examine his life, you will notice he was Mr. Rothschild's Choice as the video of the same name says. President Trump is hated by the New World Order as he does not play well with others. As the Frank Sinatra song goes, "He did it my way." Mr. Biden appears to be a clone as the ears are not quite right.

Mr. Clinton is a good example of Mr. Rothschild's choice. He was selected as a Rhodes scholar and sent to Oxford where he could be indoctrinated in the ways of the New World Order. Cecil Rhodes was one of the world's leading imperialists and advocates of socialism, eugenics and Communism. His scholarships were left to supply training for leaders to implement British world dominance. Bill Clinton was a perfect candidate because as we all know now is a sex and drug addict, and he was consumed with a lust for power. Bill and Hillary were frequent visitors to Epstein's

Orgy Island and Bohemian Grove Satanic ceremonies. Therefore, he was someone readily blackmailed. He willingly took his training, Satanic Order membership, etc. in return for sex and his god cash. (Over $100 million that we know of.). After completing scores of financial scandals, Bill went on to be the governor of the State of Arkansas, where he helped ship a lot of drugs and drug money for the CIA. Since he did such an excellent job, he got the # 1 slot and got to be placed as President with his lesbian CIA handler wife Hillary the power behind the throne. Bill and Hillary are often seen at Satanic Sex Ritual practices, where Hillary is fond of indulging in lesbian sex with the Satanic Priestess as she is one herself. You can catch the whole story on video: Revelations of a Mother Goddess by an escaped sex slave. Hillary is very well placed in the New World Order banking establishment and has some secret directorships such as American La Forge- the chemical company that made the components of Saddam Hussein's poison gas. This poison gas was then deployed in "ethnic cleansing" or mass murder of the Kurds and opposition groups to CIA henchman Saddam Hussain.

Seems like we have seen this pattern of mass extermination of large groups before under Adolph Hitler. Hitler was of course, one of the best known and most openly displayed Satanic Master. Using his occult knowledge, he channeled the Satanic consciousness directly through his mouth. Hitler's mesmerizing speeches were not his own. He was just a channel for pure evil, no more and no less, and he paid the price in nightmares for it.

I mention Adolph Hitler because the N.W.O. bankers through Prescott Bush, the grandfather of the president, financed him. Wall Street and Prescott Bush raised one-third of the money for the Nazi war machine. With his friends from Yale's Skull and Bones, a Satanic Order, Prescott Bush created the family's fortune of $1.5 million- all paid in blood. Prescott's son and grandson continued the family tradition at Yale, Skull and Bones, and the extermination of millions behind the scenes. More about the Bush family will come later.

To control a population and its economy, you need a bank. If you have ever read the Communist Manifesto by Karl Marx, you will notice that creation of a central bank is on the list. Like the first and second Bank of the United States the Federal Reserve Bank was created during top-secret meetings at Jekyll Island, Georgia. The principal architect of the Federal Reserve Bank was Max Warburg, the right-hand man of the Rothschild's and possibly a member of the Satanic 13. The Federal Reserve Bank was built as a mechanism to stabilize the economy and prevent the bank panics that the Rothschild's had in fact created over a 50-year period. The new bank was incorporated in Delaware and later the Philippines. Member banks are all N.W.O. establishment banks under the direct control of the Illuminati Brotherhood. These private banks then use the Internal Revenue Service as a collection agency and launder the money most often through Puerto Rico.

Once set up, the central bank can print money for nothing, multiply it 66 times, and then loan it back to the U.S. government at interest. Most of this money found its way back to the Bank of England and the crown, the true owner of America. But that is another story. Within 16 years, 1929, the Federal Reserve Bank flooded the market with money and then pulled open the gallows' trapdoor to hang the investors and plunge the world into the Great Depression. What a coincidence! After financing a couple of world wars, the Russian Revolution, and raising hell, all the USA's gold from Fort Knox was carried off to the Bank of England in 1968 by military convoy and left us flat broke. That was why the gold standard was abandoned in 1971. There is no more gold in Fort Knox. It is empty. Another Great Worldwide Depression will occur whenever THEY feel like it. **THEY cannot usher in a One World government until THEY destroy the one we presently have**. No one will beg for a new system while the present one is still working, so they must break it. Again, destroying society is essential to Marx's theory. We will talk more about how THEY plan to do it later. This is also happening right now!

The most useful analogy of the N.W.O. Central Banking System is to think of them as corporate raiders and doing a hostile takeover. The target country or area, like Malaysia or Japan, is first "set up" with easy money. Everybody loves almost free money, but there are strings attached. When the strings are pulled, the money is shut off and the whole house of cards falls. Everything crashes, everybody is broke, and the bankers buy everything at 5% on the dollar, yen, or Ringlet and start the cycle over again. And no one seems to catch on.

Your reaction to this scenario might be that this is only normal business cycles, and that it is impossible for any one group, even a large group, to crash an entire country, or even the whole world. First, you must remember that the power elite controls most banks, politicians, militaries, and intelligence agencies. These events are planned for years or decades, and then blamed on someone and something else. If you do not believe that this cannot be done, you need to reexamine the history of banks and stock exchanges' sting and sucker plays which were orchestrated by the great master manipulator, Nathan Rothschild. Back in 1824, Nathan Rothschild spread the rumor that the British had lost to Napoleon at the Battle of Waterloo of which he had financed both sides. He faked frantic selling, started a panic and owned England by the end of the day. Investors were not too happy to find out that Wellington won a couple of days later. But they had been hoodwinked. Just as we are being played now!

This brings us full circle to the New World Order's newest and most successful to date creation! Terrorism and bioterrorism like Covid-19. Problem Reaction Solution. Terrorism is just an extension of the Divide and Conqueror Principle. It appears that there are divisions into Communist terrorists, Arab terrorists, Nazis, Chinese, terrorists and Fascists etc. However, they are not. All these various" isms were created by the same people to do the same thing: to manipulate the target population. Always remember the #1 principle in solving any crime: follow the money!! Who do you think paid ghostwriter Karl Marx to write The Communist Manifesto? Snow White? No. A Rothschild wrote the check. Who gave Lenin $10 million in a suitcase? Wall Street bankers, like Rockefeller. Who gave the money to Hitler? Yeah, already told you that one. So, whom do you think gives money to terrorists? Yeah, you got it: N.W.O. bankers. Cannot sell bullets and guns and loan money at high interest unless you have someone to fight. Nothing in this world happens by accident. Nothing. All you must do to manipulate an ignorant public is create an "event", and everyone will jump on board. Need to invade Iraq to steal all the oil? No problem. Need an oil pipeline across Afghanistan and a way to harvest the opium? No problem. Take any war, be it The American Revolution on up. Where does all the money come from and why? Hey, it is good business! Money is made on blood. Fast-forward 200 years and look again with eyes that see. Let us look at a few events in the light! Remember the Maine, remember the Lusitania. As the villain, Elliot Carver, in the James Bond movie Tomorrow Never Dies said, "Give me a headline and I'll give you a war." No one is safe unless we vaccinate the entire world. It is for your protection just as Adolph Hitler said.

Oklahoma City. A guy named Timothy McVeigh is alleged to have blown up the Federal Reserve Building with a load of fertilizer. He is supposedly mad about Waco, Texas massacre of cult members. Does that make sense to you? The problem is that his bomb never went off. But the extremely high-tech barometric bomb the intelligence agencies planted does go off and kills dozens of people, including a lot of kids. The Feds' hastily tear down the building, bury it, and put a fence around it. Why? To discredit the Christian Militia and get guns away from the people. Cannot have a One World government if anybody has a gun. Gun confiscation is always the first step. Check out Hitler, Stalin, Mao and anyone else who has ever confiscated guns and you will see what carnage follows.

Waco, Texas. A bunch of Feds arrive with an army to serve a warrant on David Koresh. Four of them jump on the roof of the compound. One Fed climbs through the window. The three on the roof are all killed. All three are former President Clinton bodyguards. What a coincidence!! Add these three to the 140 others that the Clinton crime family already bagged and tagged. Great shooting David. I bet you stayed up for months planning that one! So, the Feds ram the building full of women and children and inject a poison gas, which then blows up. The surviving unarmed women and children fleeing from the building are gunned down with machine guns. Guess whom Janet Reno works for?

Sept 11, 2001, NYC. The Mother of all Terrorist Attacks! Around three thousand people die when two planes hit the World Trade Center, a few minutes apart, and the towers collapse. Except there were no planes. The worst terrorist attack since Pearl Harbor, if not ever! The Pentagon is hit. Another plane crashes in Pa. The alleged terrorists left evidence in their luggage in their cars. How convenient. Who thought that one up? We are told that Al Qaeda and Bin Laden did it. He says he did not. The whole country wants revenge, so the U.S. bombs the hell out of Afghanistan, chases the Taliban, and kills a lot of civilians in addition to the Taliban. A pro-oil pipeline government is installed, and heroin once again flows readily into the hands of the CIA. Lots of nasty details begin to appear a year later. Apparently, the buildings were blown from the bottom using thermite bombs which would have taken months to install. The question of who did it remains unanswered. I am guessing the Deep State.

George Bush Sr. and Bin Laden are business partners in the Carlyle Group. Clinton had refused to arrest Osama Bin Laden on several occasions, most notably in the Sudan. The Bin Laden family flies out of the USA on 9-11 in a plane, the only plane in the USA not grounded. President Bush refused to authorize investigation into 9-11. FBI and civilian warnings were ignored. The oil pipeline looks like a done deal. Preparations to invade Afghanistan were made months before 9-11. Elite US Mountain troops train for Afghanistan in June of 2001. High-level CIA directors sell short airline stock, making millions. The terrorists all entered the country legally. Three show Pensacola Naval Air Station as their home address on their drivers' licenses. The flight schools are in known CIA hangouts. We learn that the military has had "remote control" spy/reconnaissance, a year prior to 9-11. On 9-11 Florida Senators "do lunch" with Pakistani secret police, who allegedly gave Al Qaeda $100,000 cash for "the job." Pakistani secret police and CIA links are firmly set up. Bush and the Bin Laden families are still friends. Guess the alleged terrorists were all set up. And they are all still alive.

This one makes me so sick I am not going to say much more. Read it yourself in: Shadow Government, 9-11, and State Terror by Catastrophe- Bill

Clinton and 9-11. All I can say is that it looks like a false flag "event" to me. Several world leaders, such as the Italian Prime Minister, condemn it as a false flag operation and openly say we are all a bunch of idiots. And even worse more events are being planned. That is why I am writing a guide here to future events, so the public will not be fooled- again. This is how the Illuminati bankers do it. What if THEY threw a war and nobody came!

Next, we have the anthrax event. Senators and Congressmen targeted. Little old ladies die. Postal carriers get sick, people are afraid to open their mail. Take a closer look with my eyes:

The Daily Sun is hit with an anthrax letter: the photo editor dies! He is alleged to have a photo of George Bush in Skull and Bones Satanic Initiation Ceremony performing nude homosexual acts in a coffin with a frequent visitor to the White House. Feds, CIA, and the FBI hit the newspaper like Iwo Jima and tear it apart and close it down. Full National Security alert initiated for the photo and Feds search the internet and your computer for it. Do not know if they found it or not. Chinese spies blackmail Bush over the photo and demand military, scientific, and economic concessions which they get. Bush is not a happy camper.

Now, the USA is supposed to go to war with Iraq to destroy weapons of mass destruction. The Allies do not buy it. Weapons originally built with a $5 billion agricultural loan from US taxpayers, or I should say The Federal Reserve. If Saddam got thrown out, Hillary will have to find a new market for her poison gas, and George Bush and the Queen won't be getting their joint amount of $100 million oil kickback, but they would be able to just take over Iraq and set up their own gas station for Pennzoil which the Bush family owns a lot of. I guess the Queen would get her cut. What happened to Saddam's 20 suitcase nukes he got from the KGB for drugs? What about the Chinese neutron bombs there? Bill Clinton shut off our defense system for a bit, so we will never know where they are or if they ever existed in the first place.

So chemical weapons, weapons of mass destruction, HIV, West Nile Virus, and now Covid-19. What is next on the play list? Who knows?

According to Dr. Fauci round #2 will be a combination of 1918 Spanish flu and 2009 bird flu. He should know as he helped make it **AND PUT IT INTO THE VACCINE**. There will be more rounds every year until the world is subdued and everyone is vaccinated, poisoned and controlled. Violators will be terminated with extreme prejudice. The FEMA RED LIST will be activated. All these events are just that- orchestrated "events" to usher in the New World Order and a One World digital currency WITH THE Mark of the Beast. The economies of the entire world will have to be collapsed. Conservation areas are being bought in the name of the environment. It is just a coincidence they all have gold in them that can be used to back a One World Government without ever having to lift a shovel. Authors have died for this information. (Behold a Pale Horse by William Cooper.) Doctors who have cured AIDS are in prison. Authors who wrote about curing AIDS were sent to prison. Little old ladies making tea go to prison for violating the FDA.

We must therefore ask ourselves how and where in hell did, we get to this point? Where did it all begin so we can figure a way to end it. In our next chapter we will look at the grandfather of all evil Karl Marx the original intellectual whore himself. I apologize for taking such a long time to relay all the facts, but unless you understand the basics, you will never connect all the dots. The details have deliberately been made to be confusing. However, once you know them all you will see ALL current events come straight out of Karl Marx's and Adolph Hitler's playbook. Then we have a chance. If you have your enemy's playbook then you know how to defeat him.

CHAPTER 3

THE DEVIL AND KARL MARX

I RECENTLY SAW A WOMAN on Facebook holding up a sign that read "We want full Communism here now." Might I suggest to her that she should commit herself to the nearest prison and don an orange jump suit. Then be sure her captors rape and torture her ever day until she is no longer serviceable. Then someone can shoot her in the back of the head, sell her organs on the black market and bury her in a mass grave. Then she will have experienced "full Communism."

Exactly how many Americans have made makeshift rafts to escape the horrors of capitalism by seeking refuge in the benevolent land of Cuba? Zero- that is how many. How many have defected to Russia so they can live on $2 per year? Even's Stalin's daughter defected to the USA!! Guess what, it is the same deal in China. The democrats recently lost the State of Florida to Trump as they were preaching socialism to Cubans in Miami who knew better.

The man ultimately responsible for the propagation of Communism throughout the world is none other than Karl Marx. He and Frederick Engels jointly wrote the Communist Manifesto in Brussels Belgium in January of

1848. This was based on a model developed earlier by Engels. Marx's followers praise him as some sort of God, but the man himself was nothing of the sort.

While Marx claimed to be a champion of the proletariat or working man but, he never had a job himself believing it was below his dignity. He spent all his time in libraries and never even worked with the workers he wrote about. Somewhat like today's radical left who spout revolution from their mother's basement, Marx lived on money from family and friends. He therefore was often planning to move from city to city to evade the landlords, butchers, and shopkeepers he owed money to. He did receive a substantial inheritance upon the death of his wealthy German Jewish father of 6,000 gold talents, but he quickly went through it. If not for the financial support of factory owner Friedrich Engels Marx would have died in obscurity much sooner.

Karl Marx was a wild-eyed smelly revolutionary with unkempt hair and constantly covered in boils because he never bathed. His house was a shamble, and he was always disorderly and disorganized. He had a long-suffering aristocratic wife but found the time to have a son with the housekeeper. He was quarrelsome, loud, insulting, and often drunk. He seemed to have a loathing for the entire world however he considered himself a great poet and artist. His poetry was indeed excellent but morbid and reeked of suicide and love of Satan. His poems had anagrams naming the Antichrist as his hero. He himself said frequently that he was going to hell for what he had done with his life. At times he seemed demented and screaming at unknown visitors. His early poetry speaks of swords and the Antichrist. Bloggers and biographers have often wondered if he had given his soul to Satan and joined a secret cult. I personally believe he was the Antichrist of his age and had the corresponding spiritual calibration and negative karma associated with his lifestyle. His modern admirers love to gloss over his life then paint him as a great man. This is not the truth. There is a reason Marx was an atheist bent on destroying all the religions and churches of the world. Over 100-200 million people would be tortured and killed and over 40,000 churches were closed, dynamited or burned down all for the insane ravings of one madman with a black heart.

Marx was a product of his time in history. He was correct in his observation that dramatic changes in economic production and social organization inevitably create dislocation of workers. The industrial revolution was perhaps the greatest economic change in history as it displaced the feudal system before it into a wage for work system. This transition produced a new class of workers which Marx called the proletariat. The working class or proletariat were treated harshly and called the scum of the earth. Those of the working class who were unemployed and homeless were considered vagrants and could be whipped, branded or simply hanged without much fanfare. Vagrants, minstrels, actors and Gypsies were assumed to be thieves and treated accordingly. As early as 1598 King Henry VIII had 78,000 people executed. Prisons and workhouses for the poor were deplorable. Eventually the concept of transportation developed whereby prisoners were shipped to America and later to Australia to supply some service to the Crown of England. Millions of Irish was transported to the plantations of the Indies, such as Jamaica, as slaves and forcibly bred with African slaves to set a higher price on the slave market.

The writings of Voltaire, Rousseau, and Locke helped fuel the American Revolution and the French Revolution. During this period of massive change revolutions were in the air. Riots, workers' strikes, and revolt were common in the 1840s. The short-lived Paris revolt of two months may have been the first revolt orchestrated by the newly formed Communist Party. It was brutally put down.

The main theme of The Communist Manifesto is the inherent class struggle between the workers who have been used badly and disposed of by the wealthy ruling class which profits from their cheap labor.

The Communist's cure for class struggle is to foment revolution, seize all private property and means of production. Furthermore, all religions are banned as they are merely the opiate of the masses and detract from the attention of the masses from the state.

The problem with Communism is that it has no basis in reality but is a utopian pipe dream. Due to inherent human nature, it is unworkable. All utopian communities and experiments in the history of the world have failed. Even our pilgrim ancestors discovered that it does not work, but you never hear of this experiment. Only monasteries have passed the test of time therefore Communism relies on brute force, mass executions, slavery, and gulag prison camps. Dynamiting of churches, bribery, secret police, spies and any means necessary to force compliance to the Communist ideal. Therein lies the rub; Communists will infiltrate any country, any organization, spread propaganda, commit murder and all forms of treachery to advance their unholy cause. This can be seen every day in this country.

Stalin's quote "the death of one man is a tragedy, the death of millions is a statistic." The Russians killed over 100 million people. Chairman Mao may have exceeded him. The Cambodian Communist Dictator Pol Pot killed 1.5- 2 million in mass murders. Even though the Russian experiment lasted almost 100 years, they never delivered a new man, nor did Hitler produce the new man. The answer of how to create a new man with a diamond body will be given in Part 2 of the solution. It is NOT Hitler's new man.

The Communist Manifesto is certainly one of the most underread and misunderstood documents in history. Therefore, it is extremely relevant that we discuss the main points of the Communist agenda, so we have a full understanding of what the promoters of the New World Order have in mind for us.

1. Abolition of property in land and application of all rents of land to public purposes.

2. A heavy progressive or graduated income tax.

3. Abolition of all rights of inheritance.

4. Confiscation of the property of all immigrants and rebels.

5. Centralization of credit in the hands of the state, by means of a National Bank with state capital and exclusive monopoly.

6. Centralization of the means of communication and transports enhance of the state.

7. Extension of factories and instruments of production owned by the state, the bringing into cultivation of wastelands, and the improvement of the soil generally in accordance with the common plan.

8. Equal obligation of all to work. Establishment of industrial armies, especially for agriculture.

9. Combination of agriculture with manufacturing industries, gradual abolition of the distinction between town and country, by a more equitable distribution of population over the country.

10. Free education for all children in public schools. Abolition of child factory labor in its present form. Combination of education with industrial production, etc.

There should have been a #11 plank stating that the world is to be united into a New World Order government under Satan, but that was too obvious.

The very first plank of The Communist Manifesto is the abolishment of all private property and public ownership by the state. The right to own private property is enshrined in the American Bill of Rights as an inalienable right given to us by God. The confiscation of all private property by the state is a radical revolutionary idea that is unworkable and unmanageable in practice. If you have ever had a slacker of a landlord who never fixed your heating system, all winter or sprayed for the bugs in your kitchen you'd have known better. The state property owner who is 3000 miles away and does not know or care about you certainly is not going to worry about your dwelling. Look at Cuba, an entire country in need of paint. I think the truth to be self-evident. How can a central committee care for 100 million properties efficiently? They cannot! There is an old saying "a camel is a horse designed by a committee!" American government isn't any better. The IRS seized the famous brothel known as The Mustang Ranch in Nevada and quickly drove it out of business. How dumb is that?

The second plank calls for a heavy progressive income tax seldom works as those who have the most to lose will simply relocate to a low or no tax country. This is happened in the USA as corporations transferred their offices and patents and intellectual property to Ireland as it has a 10% flat tax rate. This greatly enriched Ireland at the expense of American workers. There are at least 30 offshore banking centers around the world to hide your money from the tax man. The IRS vilifies these offshore banks as they want to steal your money

The abolition of all rights of inheritance also causes all capital to flee to a safe haven like Switzerland or the Cayman Islands. The increase in capital generated by inheritance can be very substantial as homes and property are the prime storehouse of wealth for people worldwide. Inheritance capital is also a prime source for investments and the generation of new businesses. Without inheritance capital flow and the creation of new businesses would be greatly diminished if not destroyed.

Confiscation of all property of immigrants and rebels only serves to stop immigration to a country that will confiscate their property. And a rebel would be anyone who disagrees with the state therefore anyone's property could be confiscated on the grounds of disagreement with the state which is exactly what has occurred. Millions have been put in prison or executed exactly because they refused to relinquish their wealth and property to the state. In China dissidents are reeducated (tortured) in camps to divulge the location of their money. Therefore all the money laundering laws were enacted in the USA so the state can confiscate your money.

Centralization in a National Bank allows the state to control all credit and issuance of money which invariably has no gold backing and is in the control of the banking elite at interest. It also allows for the financing of world wars and the complete destruction of entire countries. Wars are not possible without financial backing as they are extremely expensive. Therefore, the best way to eliminate war is to limit or eliminate central banks. The Constitution of the United States says that the government is only responsible for the weights, measures and purity of metals such as gold and silver. It is the printing press printing paper money without any backing that allows world wars to happen and that is exactly why they were created in the United States. It also allows the state to collapse the economy whenever it feels like it so the bankers can then buy everything at bargain prices and then repeat. Central bankers have no desire to back their paper money with gold to provide stability to the government. Private banks in Switzerland and elsewhere have 100% gold backing on their deposits. The bad guys have attempted to reduce this and to create instability as that is their goal. They call gold a "barbarous relic" when in truth THEY own nearly all the world's supply and hoard it to keep it from the public. Gold is predicted to increase in value to $3,000/ ounce by next year and to $11,000 by 2025 according to Jim Richards.

Centralization of all means of communication and transportation both need tremendous infrastructure and maintenance. The larger the systems, the more difficult to keep effective management. Without competition there is no incentive to offer superior service, the customer will be damned!

Control of all factories and means of production means no competition. Little if any innovation eventually leads to extreme shortages particularly food shortages. Lines for bread in Russia could extend for several blocks if bread were available at all. Necessities became luxury items. Capitalist systems produce an abundance of affordable products in vast variety.

The combination of agriculture and industry and the abolition of towns and countries by central planning. This is the worst viable way to accomplish objectives in production. As market forces are not in operation the whole plan is a haphazard scenario and can only be kept by force if it is a miss. During the French Revolution, the bean counters guessed that there was an excess unsustainable population, therefore they slaughtered all the inhabitants of one town to make the numbers right. This is exactly what is happening now in the USA as the bad guys believe automation will reduce the work force by 70% and they want to keep everyone under control.

Education of all children by the state has already been carried out in most countries. Having state education for all youth is particularly effective for creating Hitler youth and zealots for the cause. State care of children instead of their natural parents only leads to maladjusted adults. It also disrupts the transmission of survival skills and talents that may have taken hundreds of years to develop. Destroying the family only leads to a destruction of knowledge for a productive society and the substitution of unquestioning robots. State care of children is only advocated by those who love creating bastard children with no consequences.

Karl Marx had a particularly dark view of history and the future of humanity. While it is true that life in the mid-1800s was brutish and short and 90% of the workers were without property. However not all historians share Marx's negative viewpoint. Recent scholarship published as **Liberty's Dawn: A Peoples History of the Industrial Revolution** shows many positive gains.

Marx could not have envisioned life in America 170 years later when 65% of Americans own their own homes and everyone has a car, tv and computer. An even more surprising statistic is that 6.7% of Americans are millionaires. College dropouts have created billion-dollar companies from their garages. Even a former California chicken farmer recovered $400 million from a Spanish galleon. New millionaires are created every day in America.

The bottom line is that Communism just does not work and despite any hype it never has. Even Lenin had to allow a "New Economic Policy" in 1922 and capitalism to keep the country from falling. **My favorite Lenin quote however is when he said, "people who get caught up in this really are idiots."** The only reason Communism survived at all was from help from the West and outright theft of our intellectual property. As an example, consider what would happen if someone found a $1 million dollar gold nugget on the beach and was foolish enough to give it to the state. Ideally the $1 million could be given out to a million people at the rate of $1 each. However, the cost of delivery could be 90%. That is only in theory that everyone would maybe get a cup of coffee. The reality is the Communist system is not equal as the party members live like kings with mansions, caviar and prostitutes while everyone else lives like slaves as they did before. Party members get a free apartment, vacation homes, extra pay, foreign travel, a car and the workers get an early grave. Look at Castro and you will see what I am talking about or any other Communist leader. In the capitalist scenario if an individual found $1 million, he could buy a home, have a family, and start a business. His $1 million would generate jobs for others and not be wasted on foolish schemes and projects.

In theory everyone under Communism would be the same and equally poor. The truth is the elite live like Roman Emperors and the proletariat live like the serfs and peasants they have always been. Nothing has really changed except the rhetoric. Fidel Castro liked to paint himself as a man of the people who loved his fisherman's hut. Except his parents had a 25,000-acre sugar plantation and he had a nice 75-acre home, a hunting lodge, 30,000 female sexual conquests, and $900 million in his bank account. He stole roughly 10% of the wealth of the country. Meanwhile all the workers in the fields must live on $30/month, have poor schools and no medicines despite apologists for Communism like Bernie Sanders. Everything in Cuba is falling down.

Hugo Chavez made Castro look like an amateur. He and his friends rigged his election and then stole $100 billion out of the $1 trillion in oil money that Venezuela receives annually. The peasants are starving due to price controls on food, but Chavez's daughter has $ billions in her account. So much for social justice!!

In a Bloomberg article of 2/15/2021 the headline states BANKRUPTED BY SOCIALISM: VENEZUELA CEDES CONTROL OF COMPANIES. Over 5 million people fled, and Columbia granted asylum to 1.2 million. Of the 1,322-business seized by the socialist government only 700 remain. The remainder went bankrupt. As people were starving in the streets the government ceded control back to hundreds of companies and invited private capital and profit sharing. Socialism just does not work. As Margret Thatcher once said, "The problem with socialism is that eventually you run out of other people's money."

Communism is backward thinking. Money is just a tool. Nothing more. Before closing this chapter, I will leave you with a few quotes from Wallace D. Wattles famous book The Science of Getting Rich which was published in 1910. (You can get a free copy from www.scienceofgettingrich.net)

"A person's right to life means his right to have the free and unrestricted use of all the things which may be necessary to his fullest mental, spiritual, and physical unfoldment: or, in other words, his right to be rich."

"The purpose of nature is the advancement and unfoldment of life, and everyone should have all that can contribute to the power, elegance, beauty, and richness of life. To be content with less is sinful."

As Bessie Smith sang in 1929 "Nobody knows you when you're down and out".

The bottom line is you can vote Communism in but then you must shoot your way back out.

CHAPTER 4

ENTER THE DRAGON

LEFTIST LEANING POLITICIANS HAVE TRIED to convince us that China is different from Russia and that our government needs to support China to keep the status quo against Russia. This was particularly accepted during the time that Russia invaded Afghanistan. The truth is both the Russian revolution, and the Chinese Communist revolution were financed by illuminati Wall Street bankers.

The Communist Chinese under chairman Mao were aided due to political pressure by the Council on Foreign Relations. The nationalist Chinese who were our allies against Japan were forced to return all their Lend Lease military supplies and were left defenseless against the Communist forces. This was the only occasion that Lend Lease weapons were returned. Consequently, the Communist forces were able to use captured Japanese military supplies to defeat the free nationalist forces. The nationalist forces fled to Taiwan as a government in exile and have been there ever since.

The Communist PLA considers America to be their main adversary and developed what they call the thousand talents program based on long term strategic deception. As said in the art of war deception is the first rule of warfare and with the help of the Deep State, they play it well.

There is no difference between the Communism of China and that of Russia. Just because Russia is currently playing possum posing as a capitalist country does not mean a single bureaucrat has lost their party jobs. And both countries are committed to the Marxist concept of a New World Order based on Satan with no religions allowed nor any private property. When China invaded Tibet, millions were killed, and monasteries were burned just as in Russia. The Chinese have done everything to destroy the rich ancient culture and heritage of Tibet. Like Hitler's Germany the Chinese needed breathing room.

The Communists would have never conquered China without the support of our State Department and Wall Street financial backing. Chairman Mao's great leap forward was an attempt to modernize the country and create manufacturing and a steel industry. As I have said previously economic decisions made by a committee thousands of miles away all result in disaster. 50,000 died during a great famine as Communism overtook China's prosperous agricultural communities. They were nationalized and as a result 30 to 65 million people died due to either starvation or murder by being buried alive.

China would have collapsed economically if it had not been saved again by our government. President Nixon made a great show of normalizing relations with China at the advice of globalist and CFR member Dr. Henry Kissinger. Free trade agreements were signed under the Carter, Clinton, and Bush administrations. They all jumped on board to make China a favored nation. These free trade deals resulted in multibillion dollar trade deficits and massive amounts of cash for the Chinese. The Chinese then used their cash to promote revolution all over the world including Central and South America. The Monroe Doctrine was abandoned. Both ends of the Panama Canal are controlled by the Chinese!! The Communist takeover in Venezuela resulted in crashing the economy of what once was one of the most prosperous nations. Hell bent on world domination the Communists keep selling their false utopia to the unsuspecting. Eventually however ideology collides with reality!!

The Chinese infiltration of the USA has been particularly alarming and detrimental to our way of life. The Chinese use the very freedom of our society against us to infiltrate and destroy. They have been quick to use our lax immigration laws to set up businesses and to buy out businesses. Everyone likes free money pumped into their community not realizing there are strings attached. First, China is not a free capitalist country. Chinese businesspeople are merely vassals of the PLA and a platform for spies to steal American intellectual property. And they are using their money to influence education and elections.

There are at least 500,000 Chinese students in the USA here legally. The party has paid millions in fees to universities to set up Confucius Institutes to sugarcoat life in China and to subvert gullible students to their cause. Political officers of the PLA also ensure their students are politically correct. Meanwhile thousands of organized Chinese illegally cross both the Mexican and Canadian borders estimated at 1/3 of all illegals. The Biden Administration is putting these terrorists and spies up in hotels at taxpayer expense. (And in August 2021 the Biden administration left a few billion in military equipment for use by the Taliban.) According to section 3 of the US Constitution "aiding and abetting the enemy" is treason. How many acts of treason must be committed before anyone begins to prosecute?

The bottom line is that Communist society invariably kills all creativity and innovation therefore they must steal our intellectual property at a rate estimated to be between $225 to $600 billion dollars per year. Chinese agents unsuccessfully tried to gain control of the United Nations Intellectual Property Organization. With this exception the Chinese have had remarkable success infiltrating most committees of the United Nations and placing sympathetic individuals as secretaries of state of the United Nations for the past 30 years.

As if established businesses and universities (and the Biden Administration) were not supplying enough spies, China employs 50,000 to 100,000 hackers to both disrupt communications and steal our protected intellectual property. They have made a great push to beat out the competition for 5G and to market Huawei's landlines and business machines. Consequently, the Trump administration has banned all federal agencies from using Huawei equipment as it poses a formidable threat to national security.

The money earned from trade deficits have bankrolled four of the largest banks in the world. These are the Industrial and Commercial Bank of China, Bank of China, China Construction Bank, and the Agricultural Bank of China. They are often interlocked with the major illuminati banks in New York and have been accused of money laundering and other deficiencies. Loans from these banks are used to gain concessions in South and Central America and around the world.

The Chinese have also used their funds to buy major businesses and infrastructure in the USA such as radio, TV and movie studios. The most talked about acquisition was the purchase of Smithfield Pork processing plant which controls 25% of America's pork. Having an enemy combatant controlling 25% of any American food commodity is a drastic miscalculation.

China's inroads in American universities have been large as previously noted. US colleges have received over $1 billion in donations. Harvard leads the donor list at $93.7 million dollars. This push has been started to gain American intellectual property and expertise. The case of Harvard is particularly relevant as Dr. Charles Lieber formerly of the Chemistry and Chemical Biology Department has been charged by the FBI for his participation in China's thousand talents program. He was arrested on January 28th, 2020, for making false statements concerning his involvements with China. He is considered an expert on nanotechnology, not virology. Remember this fact as the devil is in the details.

The Charles Lieber case maybe the smoking gun that solves the creation of COVID-19. This may sound like a conspiracy theory however, I will quote directly from the Department of Justice Office of Public Affairs in the Justice News of Tuesday January 28th, 2020. The heading reads Harvard University Professor and two Chinese Nationals charged in three separate China related cases. According to the Department of Justice Doctor Lieber had accepted $15,000,000 in grant funding from the National Institute of Health and the Department of Defense. These grants require the disclosure of significant foreign financial conflicts of interest, including financial support from foreign governments or foreign entities. Unbeknownst to Harvard University beginning in 2011, Lieber became a strategic scientist at Wuhan University of Technology in China and was a contractual participant in China's 1,000 talents plan from in or about 2012 to 2017. China's thousand talents plan is one of the most prominent Chinese talent recruitments plans that are designated to attract, recruit, and cultivate high level scientific talent in furtherance of China's scientific development, economic prosperity and national security. These talent programs look to lure Chinese overseas talent and foreign experts to bring their knowledge and experience to China and reward individuals for stealing proprietary information. Under the terms of Lieber's three-year thousand talents contract Wuhan University of Technology paid Lieber 50,000 US dollars per month living expenses up to 1,000,000 Chinese Jan approximately $158 thousand US dollars at the time and awarded him $1.5 million to establish a research lab at Wuhan University of Technology. In return, Lieber was bound to work for Wuhan University of Technology not less than nine months a year by declaring international cooperation projects, cultivating young teachers, and PhD students, organizing international conferences, applying for patents and publishing articles in the name of Wuhan University of Technology.

Doctor Lieber lied about his participation in the thousand talents plan and said he was never asked to participate. He was not sure how China categorized him therefore he was charged by the FBI with making false statements concerning his involvement with Communist China. Furthermore, his two research assistants were also charged. One research assistant Yangin Ye was in fact a Colonel in the People's Liberation Army of China and essentially was accused of spying and several other irregularities. The other assistant, Zaosong Zheng, stole 21 vials of biological research and attempted to smuggle them out of the United States aboard a flight destined for China. He admitted stealing the vials from a lab at Beth Israel. He was arrested for visa fraud and being an agent of a foreign government and conspiracy.

In addition to the $15 million in research money provided by the Department of Defense in setting up the Wuhan laboratory the NIH also supplied an additional $3.7 million dollars. All this financing was approved by Dr. Anthony Fauci of the NIH. I have often wondered what doctor Fauci's role has been in the creation of COVID-19. Unfortunately for Dr. Fauci he was photographed making the hand sign of the deity Baphomet. The deity Baphomet is essentially the deity of the Church of Satan. Therefore, those two fingered salutes have identified Dr. Fauci as a card-carrying Satanist. I would calibrate doctor Fauci with a spiritual calibration around 100. Therefore, I believe doctor Fauci is involved with some very heavy hitters and those of the Antichrist. Upon further investigation Dr. Fauci has bragged how his Jesuit education at the College of the Holy Cross in Worchester, New York helped him prepare for the pandemic. He has also been photographed with David Rockefeller the American architect of the New World Order and Nazi George Soros.

When you connect all the dots and discover that Bill Gates and doctor Fauci own interest in several virus patents and that Mr. Richard A. Rothschild owns the patent on the covered testing supplies (since 2015) it all starts to make sense. There is a growing movement to force Dr. Fauci to resign and/or prosecute him for covering up the whole Wuhan affair. Billions of dollars will be made by those developing a vaccine. Probably the vaccine was created years before unleashing the virus. A canine Covid vaccine was developed in 2001. Never in the history of the world has a vaccine been developed so quickly. And if we look back at the Wuhan seafood market, we must realize that it was a perfect scapegoat to launch a disease hoax because of the incredibly unsanitary conditions there. All manner of living and dead animals were slaughtered there and all their bodily fluids and excrements we are mixed in buckets. By American standards it was totally a horror story. And quite conveniently was close to the high-speed train going to Shanghai. The Chinese government deliberately suppressed the truth about the severity (and the cause) of the virus until such time as 50,000 Chinese were able to travel abroad and therefore allegedly spread the disease. Originally, whistle blowers were threatened with seven years in prison for providing western journalists with any information about the exact nature of the Covid-19 virus. The whole Covid-19 conspiracy may be even more clandestine that it appears. I smell a rat!! All smoke and mirrors. The fish market scenario appears to be just an elaborate coverup. The data suggests that 1/3 of those affected initially with Covid-19 had NO contact the seafood market. The Chinese left a trail of breadcrumbs away from the true nature of the pandemic to throw everyone off the trail. They planted another false trail about viruses escaping from a lab. I think what we have is a false flag operation within another false flag. They want you to believe there is a virus on the loose from an evil government lab in Wuhan. However, the devil is in the details. Dr. Lieber was not a virologist. He was an expert on nanotechnology. **The vaccine may be the killer, not a virus.** Will explore this in greater detail in coming chapters.

The bottom lines is that Covid is just one more plank in the planned hostile takeover of America by the Chinese. Of the half million Chinese students that are here legally we can only guess how many are military trained and only waiting for orders and arms. As early as 20 years ago caches of weapons were found hidden in California near San Francisco. However now with Democrats in power weapons can be stockpiled on military bases ready for use in the event of a national "emergency" which will be created. There are allegedly 200,000 Chinese troops on the Mexican border and 50,000 on the Canadian border just waiting. While Chinese special forces are being staged in Texas at American military bases. All they must do is put on United Nations uniforms and its fine for them to invade the USA at the request of the Biden administration. Troops may be composed of not only Chinese but Russian, Cuban, North Vietnamese and North Korean elements. And do not forget all the hundreds of thousands of illegal Chinese spies that have already crossed the Mexican border are comfortable in hotels provided by Joe Biden. The only thing preventing an outright takeover of America is the 2nd amendment. The Chinese are aware that American gun owners have 300 million weapons.

The Chinese have staged operations out of their embassies in Houston and San Francisco. The activities of 25,000-40,000 spies were discovered in Houston and that embassy was shut down. However, the San Francisco Embassy stays open to direct the movement of their military and spies. They control the "trained Marxists" known as Black Lives Matter and helped direct all the riots we have experience over the last year. All those who hate America have joined together, Communists, Nazis, Jihadists, and anarchists. There will be more riots coming as the goal of Communism is to destroy all the existing social order. Communism and Nazism love to recruit those with no future in society and give them uniforms and medals and power to destroy for a cause. Eric Hoffer made a brilliant analysis of this in his epic book **The True Believer: Thoughts on the Nature of Mass Movements.** I suggest every American read it. This is what is happening now.

American's wouldn't be so sympathetic to Communism if they understood what it is really all about. Anarchist Sergey Nechayev wrote a small paper in 1869, which he called The Catechism, which makes Marx look like a moderate. He states, "**The only form of revolution beneficial to the people is one which destroys the entire State to the roots and exterminates all the state traditions, institutions, and classes. Our task is terrible, total, universal, and merciless destruction.**"

While I hope violence is to be prevented however it would be a good idea for every American to own an AR-15 and a long-range hunting rifle in case of invasion. Committees of Safety need to be formed to prevent either Chinese or police from going house to house to confiscate guns or remove people with bogus Covid tests. Every committee of 100 should invest in a 50-caliber sniper gun for use in guerilla warfare and to harass any Chinese troop movements. Tomahawks, bayonets, and Bowie knives still work for close in work. I am sure the old Texas Rangers know how to conduct Apache style warfare.

Each state needs at least a 50,000-man National Guard or militia for use in the event of a Chinese invasion from both Mexico and Canada. Currently I am told that Chinese engineers and doctors are crossing the Mexican border to infiltrate.

For more recommendations on how to deal with the Great Reset see Mike Adams Global Reset Survival Guide. Its free at https://naturalnews.com, https://lifeinthe spirit.net or search Health Ranger and Mike Adams. Everything that is happening daily is part of the 10 Steps of Genocide. As this is the crux of the issue, I will devote a new chapter to it so you can recognize it. The bad guys cannot wait to exterminate all of us "deplorables". THEY believe automation will reduce the need for human workers by 70% so they want to prevent the masses getting out of hand and revolting.

CHAPTER 5

THE NEW WORLD ORDER

YOU MAY RECALL THAT THE Communist Manifesto believes all property should belong to the state. Owning private property is SOCIAL INEQUALITY. While the concept is antithetical to our freedom under the Constitution, the NWO continues to use stealth programs to advance their one world Communist agenda under Satan.

As a nuclear third world war confrontation has been blocked by the Galactic Confederation. (SAC nuclear missile sites were deactivated and nuclear bombs on the moon were neutralized.) The NWO decided to use pandemics and vaccines to depopulate 90% of the world. **The pandemic is a hoax, but the vaccines are not.** As the terrorism model was getting old, they decided to hijack the environmental movement and the fictitious global warming issue. Few are aware that NASA scientists have decided that the increased planetary temperatures are caused by fluctuations in solar radiation. Secondly, spiritually speaking, the Earth is ascending and heating up. The activities of man have negligible effect on this, although we would all appreciate less pollution and cleaner air. The actual affect of man's activity on the planet is a mere 3% of CO2. So why are THEY demonizing us? The NWO is deliberately holding back technology to clean the environment as this would ruin their agenda to take over the land and exterminate the population.

The NWO is using Agenda 21/2030 to confiscate or control land use in the USA with billion-dollar green urban redevelopment plans to pack the people into a confined space. Plan, develop and seize. This is called creating a ghetto and we have seen this before. **The REAL reason for this herding into urban ghettos is that 5G may only be effective for 100 meters and the population can't be controlled or exterminated if they are out of range!** That's why THEY WANT TO ELIMINATE ALL FARMERS. All that is missing is the gold arm bands with the Star of David on them. But you will not need a Star of David on your arm as the plan is to give everyone a digital tattoo with all your information. Will this be the second attempt to create the Aryan Master Race by killing everyone who does not have Aryan genes? The taxpayers get the bill like it or not. The terms HUMAN SETTLEMENS AND RELOCATIONS should send chills down your spine.

Wildlife corridors sounds very friendly until you look at a map of the proposed conservation areas and realize half of the US farmland would be gone. So where is our food supposed to come from? China? The US government already owns half the land, so there would be virtually nothing left. The Federal Government owns 90% of Nevada. As farmers are independent, out of range of 5G towers, have guns and can grow their own food it is a top priority to eliminate them.

If you read the fine print in FEMA's Resettlement plan, you will see there are 800 detention camps with gas chambers under control of UN troops. (Chinese troops). A One World BENEVOLENT GOVERNMENT sounds warm and fuzzy until you get to the FOURTH REICH part. Perhaps Hitler's or Dr. Mangala's great-grandson are not as bad as grandpa. Who knows? Let us just cut through all the flowery words and tell it like it is. The NWO Agenda 21 is a crock of shit and I will tell you why.

I was really feeling like a genius the other day as I was able to solve the global warming catastrophe in about 10 seconds. I was reading how the Swedish Navy planted 300,000 oak trees after the Napoleonic Wars in 1830 to build their ships in the future. It occurred to me that planting enough trees could absorb the CO_2 emitted by automobiles until a better solution can be implemented.

According to arborist Ben McInerney an Aleppo pine tree can absorb 50 tons of CO_2 in a year. Therefore 100 mature trees can absorb the CO_2 from 103,730 vehicles! Wow! Even less efficient trees like the Chinaberry tree can offset 7 vehicles with 10 trees on a street. If you think this cannot be implemented, you're wrong. The Indian province of Madhya Pradesh planted 66 million trees in 12 hours. A new Guinness World record beating the 50 million trees planted by Uttars Pradesh in 24 hours. Even Vietnam wants to plant 300 million trees. One farmer in Brazil and his wife planted 2 million trees by themselves. We do not need human resettlement areas. We do not all need to live in low-income housing and take the bus to nowhere as there are no jobs. For many reasons it is necessary for the population to be on the land as only humans can heal it. See Plant Spirit Reiki by Fay Johnstone. It is an unknown fact that Jesus healed the Earth on the island of Iona the sacred isle. You can do the same.

If you study history, you will realize all the current agendas proposed by the bad guys are to correct scenarios THEY implemented in the first place. At the turn of the last century the Rockefellers were busy tearing up all the trolley and rail lines so people would have to buy gas and cars. Now they want a carbon tax to fine us for their scheme. Such BS.

Hemp was once a thriving industry in the US, particularly into the 1930s. Back in the days of sail hemp was used to make rope. Although hemp has no hallucinogenic properties like its close cousin marijuana, it was outlawed. The real reason was that hemp can be made into biodiesel and would lessen the demand for Rockefeller oil. Secondly, hemp oil is reputed to cure most diseases. And even worse it would put control into the hands of farmers instead of big oil companies. It's harder to force farmers off their land and into the camps if they are prosperous. Hitler however ran ¼ of his war machine on biodiesel made from hemp. Buts that is ok. Henry Ford himself made a car that not only ran on biodiesel from hemp but the car itself was made from a plastic like material that was strong as steel made from hemp.

The problems of the internal combustion engine have been solved. The first car to run on saltwater THE QUANT, uses an ionic fluid (saline) to power 4 electric motors. Its top speed is 236 miles per hour. The nanoflowcell was unveiled in Geneva in 2014. And it does 0-60 in 5 seconds. The Quant is still a concept car now and is not in production, but the future is here. There is no need to exterminate humans to reduce emissions!!

The whole concept of overpopulation is a myth as far as America is concerned. America has enough land to give every citizen a square mile. The Federal government owns half the land and the purpose of this is to make land scarce and force people into cities and drives up prices. This then requires a mortgage from a bank that generates interest for 30 years. States like California have building codes with 78,000 laws. This is to create homelessness. Homeless people will be the first ones put on the bus to the camps as no one will miss them. That is how it works.

Thomas Jefferson bought the Louisiana Purchase of 827,000 square miles of land in 1803 for $15 million. Jefferson wanted to expand liberty. That was the goal of our founding Fathers, that every man could be his own master. The Green Agenda is to make every man a slave to the state.

The Environment Protection Agency has billions in its cleanup fund but never cleans up anything. If the environment were cleaned up then there would be no excuse for stealing the land. A product called Perfect Science Waters LLC has 70 plus formulas to clean anything from nuclear waste to sewage. The formulas can turn a swimming pool of sewage into harmless organic solids overnight. An acre of nuclear contaminated land can be cleaned for a few hundred dollars. A manufacturing plant once existed in Istanbul, Turkey as part of a joint government project. (Unfortunately, it was destroyed in an earthquake, but there are several other plants.) The Turkish government made an experiment to see if the Sea of Marmara could be cleaned. This is a saltwater inland sea found just below Istanbul about half the size of Lake Erie. A few tankers of Perfect Science Water cleaned it up overnight. Everything you have ever been told about water and pollution is a lie. A few chapters on water will be included in Part II as knowing its true characteristics and how it is affected are major keys to good health.

CHAPTER 6

THE DEEP STATE'S DECEPTIONS

THERE ARE 100S OF BOOKS about the Deep State, but unfortunately not all the dots are connected to show the big picture of deception. Therefore, I will try to provide the missing links and the reader can continue to research on their own.

The Renaissance writer Machiavelli wrote his famous tome <u>THE PRINCE</u> in 1513. He wrote that "one who deceives will always find those who allow themselves to be deceived."

The Deep State is merely the extension, or the tentacles of the money pyramid discussed earlier. At the top we have various alien beings in league with the Illuminati or Black Nobility (Satanic 13).

Two world wars were orchestrated to create a public outcry for world peace. WWI, although horrific enough, did not bring acceptance of the League of Nations. Therefore, WWII was financed at the expense of 100 million lives lost to try again for the Satanic front known as The United Nations.

Again, it was constructed on the site of an old slaughterhouse to have the proper negative energy. Once it was set up the problem of destroying the sovereignty of the USA began in earnest.

The military expenditures for WWII put millions into the coffers of Wall Street. The cold war with Russia generated billions in nuclear defense. The cost of building and keeping our nuclear defense system of 1,650 ICBMS and 160 tactical nukes is estimated to cost $1.2 trillion over their projected utility to 2046. However, this only accounts for 6% of the defense budget. Ever wonder why we did not have a WWIII nuclear war? According to the former director of the Israeli space program Haim Eshed, in his book THE UNIVERSE BEYOND THE HORIZON, he reveals our contact with the Galactic Federation for years. Humanity is not ready for full disclosure. General Eshed said that the extraterrestrials have prevented nuclear war many times. The Galactic Federation shut down Maelstrom Air Force Base in Montana with red glowing UFOs. A mysterious beam of light shut down the RAF in Bentwaters, UK. Lastly when the Deep State tried to explode a nuclear weapon on the moon, they destroyed the weapon.

So why are we spending $1.2 trillion on nukes if nuclear war is out-lawed in the solar system? The bottom line is that there is money to be made and the plan is to bankrupt the USA. Vietnam cost 55,000 lives and $168 million which would be about $8 trillion in todays dollars. Afghanistan was about $2.4 Billion with little to show for it. Oil pipeline deals were made with the Chinese and safely run a billion-dollar gold project. Also, copper, oil and gas all protected by the US military. Afghanistan may become the mining center of the world with $1 trillion in natural resource deposits. So, the way the system works is that the taxpayer forks the bill, the military which then secures resources for Wall Street and the Chinese businesses, with nothing returned to American citizens. Our troops bleed to enrich our enemies.

Astronomical bills are spent for defense such as the new Zumwalt destroyer at a cost of $4.24 billion each. And the F-35 fighter planes which cost $1.5 billion for 10 over their 55-year lifespan.

The purpose of our military adventures is to obtain raw materials for Wall Street companies, remove local resistance to foreign control and to bankrupt the USA.

Brigadier General Smedley Butler said it best in War is a Racket: "I helped make Mexico, especially Tampico, safe for American oil interests in 1914. I helped make Haiti and Cuba a decent place for the National City Bank boys to collect revenues in. I helped in the raping of half a dozen Central American republics for the benefits of Wall Street. The record of racketeering is long. I helped purify Nicaragua for the international banking house of Brown brothers in 1909-1912. I brought light to the Dominican Republic for American sugar interests in 1916. In China I helped to see to it that Standard Oil went its way unmolested."

To carry out these budget goals 1,000s of lobbyists descend upon our elected officials like swarms of locusts. Campaign contributions of millions of dollars, lucrative second careers for those who help get their agenda passed and funded.

Silicon Valley has benefitted tremendously from the growth of the military-industrial complex as the military needs their guidance systems, drones, satellite communications and super computers. The intelligence services can spy on anyone anytime anywhere. Your emails and cellphones can be recorded for data mining and stored for decades. Read Edward Snowden's revelation about our agencies spying on the US. Snowden said the ability to spy on US citizenry is **TURNKEY TYRANY** in the wrong hands. As our elected officials are not in control, I can assure you this capability is in the wrong hands. The FBI and CIA have even spied on our President Trump to discredit him and illegally remove him from office with fictitious charges of collusion with Russia.

Our internet services are also part of The Deep State. Facebook, YouTube, Google can not only censor your comments, block conservative news, but can redirect your searches to shape your opinions. Such is the power of redirection that it can influence an election by 10% for which ever candidate they choose. Basically, this spells an end to democracy.

Ever wonder why all the news is fake news? Amazingly simple. The bad guys own them all. The CIA owns up to 40% of some newspapers, has operatives on the executive boards of all major newspapers and tv channels. The military has Hollywood liaison officers to be sure they show the military in a positive light. The Chinese have gotten into Hollywood as well so they can put a positive spin on Communism in China. Hollywood is a hotbed of Satanic activity.

There are approximately 22 million state, federal, and local government employees. 2.1 million are federal employees. Very few of these employees are elected. There are no term limits except possible 30-year retirement. As these employees remain during the terms of several presidents there is little control over them. They can rule by decree from their agencies. Some of the worst ones are political appointees with no skills, but loyal to their party. 6,000 of Obama's Army are still around to undercut the aims of President Trump or whomever they are told to sabotage.

CHAPTER 7

THE SECRET GOVERNMENT

THE PREFERRED METHOD IN SOLVING a crime is by following the money. Bill Gates may or may not have killed 100,000s in Africa and India. We may never know. However, we can be sure Bill Gates would make billions on a COVID-19 vaccine if he were the sole owner. As I have said there are many layers to this story.

Another crime is who gets the money if grandpa and grandma die? When anyone on Social Security dies Social Security stops paying. All the money a person put into it just vanishes like the morning dew. If everyone in the family dies, then all assets revert to the state after banks take their damn sweet time getting interest. Remember Swiss banks after the holocaust.

Most Americans ASSUME Social Security and all the other alphabet soup agencies from the Federal Reserve, IRS, **Center for Disease Control** and FBI are actual government agencies. They are not. They are ALL private corporations owned by the Rothschild family and friends. (Aka the Illuminati, NWO, Satanists, Deep State or 4th Reich- take your pick of a label.) Therefore, after the medical and pharmaceutical industry make their money which can run into the $100,000s the money is forfeited. (The Rockefeller crime families are alleged to own 65% of the medical and pharmaceutical industry.) The bad guys set up accounts in your name the day you are born and can collect as much as a $1 million per person when you die with what is called "dead peasants insurance." The family of the deceased gets nothing. In the event all family members die all assets go to the state. The state has a vested financial interest in killing you, preferably just when you retire and start withdrawing a pension. Those who are labeled "over consumers" are the new pariah of the far left. It is ok if the billionaires who scold us have 15 cars, a helicopter and a $100 million yacht, but WE should take the train to save energy and save the planet. When Middle class folks become "enemies of the state" heads will roll. Those who hide their assets for confiscation by the state are labeled tax protestors and are shamed by the IRS. THEY have the same mindset as officials in Communist China who torture those who do not give their assets to the state and put them in mental hospitals. Those who are not "good citizens" are labeled mentally defective. Those smart enough to protect their assets offshore are accused of money laundering in offshore tax havens. The truth is THEY want to confiscate your money in the event of a takeover so you will be powerless to stop THEM.

Knowing all this President Trump made a surprise counterattack and NATIONALIZED THE FEDERAL RESERVE. The FED and the much hated and illegal IRS would have been gone by election time 2020 if all went well. But the election was stolen. The whole COVID-19 scheme to destroy the economy and the lives of all Americans could have blown up in the faces of the Deep State. They couldn't let that happen.

Regardless of the true origins of COVID-19 I hope every American realizes that any pandemic, real or imagined is a direct threat to the freedoms and Constitutional liberties of all. Everything about this pandemic is fishy!! Three pandemic drills were held preceding the outbreak. August 15th the DHS simulates a Flu Pandemic drill called "Crimson Contagion Exercise". Sept. 15th China's PLA Army runs a Coronavirus drill in Wuhan. Oct. 15 Bill Gates, John Hopkins University, World Economic Forum run a Coronavirus

simulation that kills 65 million virtual people. (www.johnmichaelchambers)
The FBI now wants to tap your email. H.R. 6666 (TRACE ACT) (Satanists
like to sign their work!!) has been introduced into the house by over 40
Democrats to create individual mobile health units to come to your home.
This may sound benevolent but if these units come with the Sheriff and can
drag you away without any due process, we have a major breach of privacy
and freedom. And of course, we need to let the UN take over the country to
protect us all.

Benjamin Franklin once said that "Those who would give up essential
Liberty to purchase a little temporary safety deserve neither Liberty nor
Safety." Our essential Liberties have been eroding steadily for the last 100
years with the biggest push over the last 20 with secret treaties and executive
orders. We need to get back on track, drain the swamp, and delete hundreds
of executive orders that threaten our personal freedoms and the sovereignty
of our beloved country. It is imperative we take a closer look at some of
America's dirty little secrets that most Americans are unaware of in the hopes
that the visions our Founding Fathers had for this country remain alive.

We all hold the American Constitution as a sacred document. However,
it was suspended prior to WWII and has never been put back into effect.
Although judges pay it lip service it is long gone. The system of justice we have
now is something of a wartime maritime prize court. If you are observant,
you'll notice the American flag has gold fringes around it signifying it is a
maritime court. The President has the power to suspend the Constitution
during an emergency. Therefore, he has the power to reinstate it.

The President (the elected one), a dozen state governors, and FEMA
have the executive authority to execute anyone deemed to be a threat to the
country. As the exact nature of a threat is not specified: it is open to interpre-
tation. In the event the Deep State plans to take over the country **FEMA has
a "RED LIST"** of all protestors and patriots who might object. Those on the
list are to be rounded up for either slave labor or extermination in the camps.

The greatest threat to our freedoms is that of the Deep State itself. Our elected officials in Washington DON'T control the country. Most Americans have never heard of COG or Continuity of Government. The COG duplicates all elected officials and has the same titles as "Mr. President", "Mr. Vice President", etc. Their identities are classified, and they rule from bomb hardened underground bunkers the size of an ordinary city. The elected President and officials do not have access to their plans. There are 20 secret classifications ABOVE THE ELECTED PRESIDENT. The elected officials are out of the loop as what the 850,000 minions of the Deep State are doing. As American troops are not authorized to interfere with domestic issues the Deep State has built up a huge army of police, assault vehicles, tanks and foreign troops to use in the event of an "emergency." Executive orders call for the use of millions of Chinese and UN troops if the populace should ever get out of hand and revolt. This is where the plot thickens and is the reason we must guard our freedoms vigorously. The devil is in the details.

There are very, very valid reasons we all must protect our second amendment rights, right to privacy in our phones and emails, and never never allow medical "police" to have the authority to enter our homes and take us away. You may be naive and think this can't happen here, but it already has been tested. On July 15th, 2020, the Arkansas National Guard transported Covid positive people to a medical facility by order of the governor. Covid tests are extremely easy to manipulate and make 100% positive. Then everyone ends up on the bus to the camps. If we ever give our power away it will surely be abused. The "Powers that Be" or "masters of the universe" have told us in print exactly what they have planned for us, but few have eyes that see or ears that hear. Many Americans can see the writing on the wall and gun sales are up by 40%. 100 million Americans own guns. Total gun ownership in American is estimated to be 393 million firearms. Americans are therefore the largest unofficial army in the world. Even the Chinese have only 2.5 million soldiers. If we preserve the 2nd amendment, they will have trouble getting everyone on the bus. Prior to the Revolutionary War patriots formed Committees of Safety to rush to the aid of any patriot who was being unjustly persecuted by the British. We need to do the same. We need to follow the precedents of our founding fathers.

The Bible tells us that the devil has a silver tongue. The bad guys are ALWAYS trying to sell us a One World (Communist) Government (based on Satan) for our own good and the ecology of the planet. They are not shy about putting their plans into print as they realize few people read anymore. The U.N. Agenda 21 document, written in 1992 calls for collective action and the relinquishment of sovereignty and personal freedom. It says our over consumptive lifestyle is unsustainable. It appears that the estimate was total bullshit. However, Mikhail Gorbachev went on record saying that a 90% reduction in human population would be good for the environment. The GLOBAL 2000 REPORT states that population should be CULLED BY 100 MILLION BY 2050. Pretty scary stuff all in print for public view. The Georgia Guidestones is less generous saying we need to keep global population at 500 million. So, the big hairy question is how do the bad guys plan to cull the population? And when? Creating plagues is the most cost-effective solution across the board as it kills everyone and doesn't damage property. Creating a WWIII was considered impractical as if you plan to kill everyone there is no one left to pay the bill. A batch of plague on the other hand can be whipped up for the cost of a 6 pack of beer. I believe therefore that the COVID-19 pandemic is a phase one TEST for martial law to perfect the numbers and identify weaknesses in the plan. Phase Two may be much more effective and fatal. The Delta variant may have the 1918 Spanish Flu and the Avian Flu in it. We shall see what plagues roll off the assembly line next year. The death toll in August 2021 has already been excessive. We the people need to devise a plan to put a wrench into phase 2 as the lives of 50-100 million Americans are at stake. People are dying so fast in Florida that funeral homes must rent refrigerated trucks to hold the excess bodies.

Culling humanity has a few technical issues and logistical supply problems. The first issue is how do you get everyone on the bus? (Or cattle car?) Well, you tell them they are infected and it's for their own good and the welfare of humanity. Then you lie your ass off. Same old Nazi lie. COVID-19 test kits were either defective 80% of the time or were preloaded to test positive. In Dar Es Salaam, President John Magufuli of Tanzania had his security forces secretly send samples from a goat, a sheep, and a pawpaw for COVID-19 testing. The goat and the pawpaw tested positive. Misleading the public with disinformation is a cornerstone of intelligence work. The bigger the lie the better. He plans to use traditional herbal remedies for the problem and will have nothing to do with the Colonial World Health Organization.

As asymptomatic people may refuse to get on the bus, the military has a plan to make everyone sick and enable tracking. We don't know exactly where all of the $38 billion in black ops money goes but a portion of it goes to chemtrail spraying. This is a much larger operation than you have ever imagined. Chemtrails are constantly purported to be a conspiracy theory, however many thousands of pages of documentation can be found for those who care to look. You can be sure that if the government aggressively claims a conspiracy theory, then it is a fact like UFOs. I found <u>Chemtrails Exposed:</u> <u>The New Manhattan Project</u> 2nd edition by Peter R. Kirby to be a very readable and extensively well documented book.

The Shadow government will never reveal its clandestine activities nor its black budget. However, whistle blowers do post photos and videos of the secret chemtrail fleet on the internet all the time.

Author Peter Kirby begins with the roots of the project with the famous Flying Tigers in WWII fighting the Japanese. The post-war fleet grew into the CIAs Air Asia and Air America running drugs and guns with a few passengers as cover. The Air America fleet of planes was so extensive it out-numbered the US commercial airlines. Ownership of the fleet was changed periodically, and extensive use was made of refurbished junkyard planes with no hull numbers or markings. The thousands of converted KC-135 tanker jets used are untraceable and above the secret clearance level of the elected presidents. The chemtrails are sprayed daily all over the world allegedly for weather modification to save the world from global warming. However, the deadly cocktail of aluminum and barium could kill all the plankton in the world's oceans, thereby destroying our oxygen and life support systems.

The aluminum in the spray is a conductor for massive amounts of energy broadcast into the atmosphere by HAARP stations around the world. We're talking about the energy equivalent of a atomic bomb. What this energy will do to the environment and the ozone layer is unpredictable. It may lead to an extinction level event when used for military offensive applications controlling the weather.

All of the above is scary enough but the buildup of toxic aluminum and barium in the soil, water, and our bodies is an immediate threat to our existence.

As said previously the goal of the shadow government is to cull 90% of the world's population. Having control of the world's weather is one way to starve any targeted population by turning their land into dither a desert or by flooding it with hurricanes. Either way works to destroy.

It is a challenging task to determine what level of toxicity of aluminum and barium will be needed to kill populations on demand, but my best guess is 10 more years of vaccinations and chemtrails are required. Then switch on 100G bursts of energy from cell phone towers and the target population will be dead in 1-2 hours. I believe that is the plan and why Agenda 21 wants to get everyone packed densely into cities.

In the Art of War if you know the enemy's plan you can defeat them. Continuous use of EMF blockers and equipment will give you 99% protection. Constant detoxification of the body will prevent the buildup necessary to kill you. It is wise to consider being healthy as a subservice activity. Being healthy will throw a wrench into the NWO holocaust plan. That is why I have come forward at this time as I have seen all this before.

The second logistical problem is rounding everyone up. Just send in the medical "police" or SWAT teams and take everyone to a football stadium nearby for holding until everyone can be processed. The bad guys have been very liberal in funding sports complexes. There are stadiums in nearly every city. You did not really think the bad guys were sports fans, did you? FEMA is always having drills for "national emergencies" (REX-84 drills). When they did respond to a real emergency as in hurricane Katrina, they really sucked at it. (The Coast Guard was tremendous however!)

The third logistical problem is how do you get rid of the bodies? One of America's dirties little secrets is that FEMA controls 800 "detention camps" THEY DON'T LIKE TO USE THE TERM DEATH CAMPS. The camps are mostly of WWII vintage originally built to house German POWs and Neissi Japanese. They are all fully functional and manned. The lights are on. The average camp can hold 20,000 prisoners. Some 45,000. The largest facilities are in Alaska and can hold an estimated 500,000 and 2 million prisoners, respectively. The locations of these concentration camps are published in a volume by Sam Adams entitled: <u>Understanding and Surviving Martial Law</u>. I bought my copy from <u>www.ToolsForFreedom.com</u>. Therefore, we are talking about a minimum capacity of 18.5 million that we know about. Every large military reservation has unknown capacity as do regional airports. They are also linked to Federal prisons and even the Canadian military. And yes even our friendly Canadians have camps also and 50,000 Chinese troops already there. Therefore about 5 rounds of extermination are needed to cull the projected 100 million American citizens.

Now for the bad news. All these camps are built on the Nazi model. They have gas chambers, (and a recent delivery of 5 tons of hydrogen cyanide) incinerators, 500,000 plastic coffins, and guillotines. FEMA is also alleged to have 400 million rounds of .22 caliber ammunition. Obviously, this would be enough to put 2 rounds Into the back of 200 million heads. Not to be outdone all new prisons are constructed to be airtight so all the prisoners can be gassed at will. It took me a while to figure out why FEMA would want 1000s of guillotines but then I realized that the average brain has about $2,000 worth of Ormus minerals. We are talking about gold, platinum, silver, iridium and rhodium. The only question that remains is whether the brain is served as a soup, as chilled tripe or reduced to powder before it is sold. Due to the high demand for black-market organs, you can count on your organs being removed while you are still alive. Probably without anesthetic as that is the Nazi way. After all you are only a "useless eater" to the 4th Reich. So, you see the original Nazi model is much improved. All of this is <u>only one pen stroke away</u> when THEY feel they can get away with it. Everything is in place. The question remains what are you going to do about it? If we do nothing, then heads will roll.

It is possible that the bad guys never saw the I AM AMERICA ATLAS map by Lori Toye and that the COG was built near the Yellowstone Super Volcano? Are they arrogant enough to believe they can survive in their underground bunkers, Moon bases or the military bases on Mars? Or perhaps when the first 100-foot wave crashes into the East Coast they'll all be under water in Washington DC. I doubt it. However, we do not know the timing of the coming Earth changes or the timetable of their plans. One good solar flare of 40% of the Sun's volume could certainly knock out the whole million satellite control system. Satellites will be raining down on Earth like so much burnt confetti. We ONLY know that a pandemic is the most likely scenario to cull the proposed 100 million people. When the ascension and the "desert days" will begin only God knows the hour.

Those of you who think you can live off the grid or shoot your way out are sadly mistaken. Given the high state of technology the bad guys control the odds are not in your favor. Every home in America has already been pre-located by GPS satellite technology right to your front door so the bad guys can watch as the SWAT teams or UN troops break down your door. The ecology loving masters of the universe who want to protect the environment will be the first to poison all game and fish so rebels cannot live off the land. Lyme disease was not an accident either. It was put there for a reason. It would be impossible for patriot groups to form for attack if everyone has a locator chip or smart dots giving their position to the UN troops so they can drop a drone on them. So, what to do?

As said in the <u>Handbook for the New Paradigm</u> (2), "Every reactive scenario has been dissected to the cellular level and restrictive actions planned for each of them. You are faced with the possibility of your extinction unless you can make a cosmic leap to a level of creative imagination that will completely nullify those plans." The bad guys never envisioned enlightened masters creating a new man immune to their tyranny.

CHAPTER 8

COVID-19 THE TROJAN HORSE TO ENSLAVE HUMANITY

FORMER NY TIMES REPORTER ALEX Berenson has written a timely fact filled expose on the real data of the pandemic. His report entitled <u>Unreported Truths about Covid-19 and Lockdowns</u> has been an enormous success. He states unequivocally that the fake news media has been preaching for TEAM APOCALIPSE and is nothing more than panic porn. Covid-19 is barely a category I on the severity index as 999/1,000 survive. Not like the Spanish flu at 1/50. Computer models were eventually downgraded by 96% but the media kept beating the drum for lockdowns.

I must add that the models used to predict Covid-19 lethality were pure science fiction. The computer models used were "in solitum" or to translate med-speak into common language they just made shit up.

After a review of the data, it is clear that lockdowns, masks, and social distancing are ineffective and junk science mandated for political approval ratings and more sinister ends. Social distancing makes biometric scanning easier. Masks can cause illness and deaths. The young are not at risk at all as only 1 child in a million might die from the flu. Why were all the schools shut down? And why were 50 million Americans unemployed? The numbers are no worse than smoking deaths or accidental overdoses. To add to this travesty, the old and fragile over 85 years old, those most at risk were often abandoned!! Nursing home deaths accounted for 40-50% of all fatalities. Half of those admitted to nursing home die within 5 months so this inflates the severity of the statistics and point to a huge gap in longevity care. We will attempt to fill in these gaps in medical knowledge in Part II. I have met 85-year-olds who were not only vibrantly alive, but in 1960s terminology I would define as cool and hip. You may want to hear the secret of an 85-year-old college disc jockey. As we say in Siddha yoga "death is a grave mistake!!

Scientifically speaking masks, lockdowns and social distancing are useless. Masks can create CO_2 issues. It is unlikely any virus is even contagious. Bacteria can be a problem however but wearing a mask can lead to bacterial infection and pneumonia. All the alleged counter measures to fight the pandemic may kill more than the flu itself. But the mother of all pandemic panic porn is that we will never be safe until the whole world is vaccinated. But in August 2021 the CDC said that vaccines won't keep anyone from being infected. Wow. Therefore, some light needs to be shed on the real inside story of vaccines.

We are being led down the primrose path about the necessity of vaccines to stop the Covid-19 pandemic. This is complete propaganda and following Hitler's model of taking care of us "for our own safety." And Goebbels' tactic of creating fear in the masses. As Joseph Goebbels said at Nuremburg, "if you repeat a lie often enough everyone will believe it". This is one of the Rules for Radicals. The controlled media regurgitates more panic porn daily despite the facts. You will NEVER hear about the **1968 Children's Vaccine Protection Act or Vaccine Damage Court**. How about millions of doses of vaccine contaminated by animal viruses during the cell culture process? Anti-Vaxers are labeled sociopaths who do not care about others. Anti-vaxxers are even label a threat to national security. They are enemies of the state of the New World Order. Unfortunately, the effectiveness of vaccines is highly overrated, and the associated dangers are swept under the rug.

Dr. Judy Mikovits and Kent Heckenlively, JD reveal the darker side of vaccines in their book entitled: **Plague of Corruption**. The reason for medical collusion is simple. As the old Elizabethan saying goes, "If it prosper, none dare call it treason."

Much like bank failures, vaccine failures are too big to fail. The British government estimates a total expenditure of L 12 billion pounds on vaccines. Great Britain has a population of 66 million while the USA has a population of 328 million. Therefore, we are talking about $83 billion for all USA vaccinations for one year. And then there is the rest of the world, which we cannot even estimate. If a tainted vaccine infects 100 million people, causes autism in 1/32 cases, chronic fatigue in millions and a few thousand deaths, brings out latent HIV, creates Epstein Barr, it is considered an acceptable loss to THEM. They made their money. You might not consider your own autistic child as mere collateral damage for the collective good. Vaccine companies have paid out $600 million in punitive damages but that will not bring back your child.

Scientists who refuse to cover up incriminating data have been subjected to surveillance, police raids, firing and alleged suicides. If a scientist or lab worker refuses to tow the company line, they may be found floating in a lake with a gunshot to the chest like Dr. Jeff Bradstreet. Dr. Timothy Cunningham's body floated up in the Chattahoochee River in the spring. Are you starting to get the big picture?

Vaccine companies would prefer that the public does not know what is in their vaccines or how they are made. As vaccines are made in animal cell cultures such as mice brains, monkeys, dogs, cows, pigs, chicken eggs etc. If 100,000 doses of vaccine are tainted, they would rather cover up that fact and pass the vaccine on and write the deaths off as an acceptable loss.

Unfortunately, some conditions caused by vaccines may not show up for 60 years and be quite untraceable back to the manufacturer. Vaccines LOWER immunity. They would prefer you do not ask any embarrassing questions and there is no such thing as follow up on vaccine effectiveness. It is a shot in the dark. No one has the slightest idea of what long term side effects of the new and experimental MRNA technology. I predict mass deaths to the order of 25% in some elderly populations after 2 years which I am sure is their plan. Judy Mikovits is predicting 50 million deaths in 1-3 years. It may reach 100 million. Who knows? And Congress has removed all liability from themselves and the manufacturers. You can't sue anyone for damages. That means it is going to be bad!!

Lastly, we must visit our old friend Dr. Vernon Coleman who has written a hard-hitting expose of the vaccine industry. His book is appropriately titled: **Anyone Who Tells You Vaccines Are Safe and Effective is Lying**. I think the title says it all. He chronicles the various vaccines and relates the hazards. It is hard to get compensation figures but for example the British government paid out between L 10,000-20,000 pounds each for Whooping cough vaccine damaged children. The annual compensation for the USA may exceed $100 million dollars, but this is an acceptable loss. Vaccine companies do their best to silence big claims as if everyone got L 2.75 million pounds for brain damage then there would be no profits. Thousands of big claims would bankrupt a company or severely embarrass the government in question. Therefore, the aforementioned case took 26 years to settle. Few parents have the resources to fight that long.

Jim Mars has reminded us in his book The Trillion Dollar Conspiracy that the fox is guarding the henhouse. At the present time it is legal for government workers to be involved in serious conflicts of interest, if not outright conspiracy. He cited the case of the former Center for Disease Control chief Dr. Julie Gerberding retiring from public service and becoming president of Merck's vaccine division. She now controls $5 billion. I am sure her salary is very lucrative.

The bottom line is that doctors get paid to administer vaccines. They get free trips, speaking fees, perks, and in the UK about L 20,000-L 50,000 British pounds to inject everyone. And doctors blackmail patients into getting vaccines. Well, it is a new Mercedes every year. What more can I say?

Now we must tackle the real reason for the Covid Vaccine Death Cult. As they say on TV- but wait there is more. Everyone concerned about the NWO using Covid-19 as the Trojan horse to bring in the Satanic Great Reset and the Mark of the Beast needs to see Celeste Solum's video **FORMER FEMA AGENT REVEALS WHAT COULD BE IN THE COVID VACCINE.** It is available at www.toolsforfreedom.com . The Bots, Borgs, and Humans Welcome You to 2025. This video explains in detail how the population can be reduced to a mere 99 million by 2025 if the NWO plans are fully implemented.

The vaccine is full of nanoparticle and hydrogel that are interactive and can cross the brain barrier to affect your emotions. Think happy robot. Claus Schwab says that in the future you will own nothing, and you'll be happy about it. I guess that is what the little micro motors chewing at your brain are for! The spike protein used is hollow and can carry a payload of toxins, poisons, viruses, fungus and even explosives. Even Satanic curses and other elements like demons. Wow! These bioweapons were developed by Plum Island Biowarfare in Manhattan and of course the Wuhan Institute of Virology. I hope the explosives in the brain won't be as dramatic as the exploding brains in the movie The Kingsman 2, or the exploding collars in Suicide Squad, but we'll see.

The components of the vaccine consist of aborted male fetal cells which send fear like a homeopathic tincture. Then there are the viruses from the ever-popular bat, civets, pangolins snakes, Coronaviruses, MERS, SARS other SARS -lile viruses and HIV. There may be as many as 21 other different elements added. Needless to say, all these ingredients didn't jump into the vaccine by themselves and took decades to develop. The whole infected bat fish market theory was just a cover up for the vaccine and 5G to activate it.

Those who are vaccinated can be tagged with an enzyme called Luciferase which shows up under a black light with your number just like a high-tech Auschwitz. Yup. Its named after Lucifer. Those who are vaccinated have 8x the risk of dying over those who are unvaccinated. 62% of fatalities are in those who are vaccinated. 82% of pregnant women vaccinated in the first trimester have spontaneous abortions. Just the deaths of the unborn may total 3.3 million.

However, vaccine manufacturers will only admit to a few deaths out of 20-30 million. Newsmax even carried the story of a 13-year-old Michigan boy named Jacob Clynick who died within hours of having his Pfizer vaccine on July 4th, 2021. Or Tim Zook a nurse who also succumbed. Several nurses have died from their shots. The Vaccine Injury Reporting System has allegedly deleted 150,000 vaccine deaths and only admits to 10,000. Just pregnant women alone may account for 3 million deaths as 82% of pregnant women have spontaneous abortions if they have received the shot in the first or second trimester. Even breastfeeding your infant after receiving a shot can result in the death of your baby. (When Japan stopped giving infants shots sudden infant death syndrome stopped.) And then there is the rest of the world getting shots. The death toll will be in the tens of millions.

The bottom line is the vaccine is built to be interactive with your brain and control you and even your dreams so you will dream the New World Order into existence and your soul is transferred to alien masters never to return to God.

How long will it take? How many shots? Well, the goal to eliminate or sterilize the population is by 2025. 50 million deaths are projected in round one in the USA. They make it all sound so warm and fuzzy until you look under the hood. Population stabilizations means mass genocide. Income equality means everybody is a poor Communist zombie robot doing the bidding of the powers that be. One World. One Health. One Bank. And one World under Satanic control.

Your friends may call you a conspiracy theorist or an antivaxxer as I was recently called. Resistance to being vaccinated has a historical precedent. Read the historical perspective in **Bodily Matters: The Anti-Vaccination Movement in England 1853-1907**.

The bad guys understand there will be resistance within the population and have a plan. Recently White House press secretary Jen Psaki let it slip that there will be a **Covid Vaccination Strike force.** Strike force is a military term for going door to door and neutralizing (killing) the inhabitants. Whether everyone is to be killed, vaccinated, or moved to a FEMA camp and then killed is a matter of speculation.

This doesn't sound as warm and fuzzy as "Volunteer Health Ambassador" as is currently being geared up in Lake County, Illinois. Fortunately, we have obtained a copy of their script outlining their disregard for private property, illegal solicitation, and impersonating health department officials. If allowed in to question citizens about their vaccine status they will record who hasn't been vaccinated and encourage them to get vaccinated for the public good. Their script makes it sound like they are on a noble cause, not working for Satan. However, they are instructed to trespass, and lie to everyone. If asked about vaccine safety, they are to say that side effects are proof that the vaccine is working. Does that include the side effect of death? How about massive brain hemorrhage? The July 5th issue of The New American Magazine has an extensive list of side effects on page 13. There are over 30 bleeding issues alone. Bleeding randomly through the skin sounds like welcome to the Zombie Apocalypse to me. (You can order a copy online for $1.25.) Therefore, I have coined the term **Blue Assassins** for these volunteers. Let the truth be told.

As the goal of Covid vaccination is depopulation and sterilization of our citizens it is imperative to resist by all legal means these unConstitutional intrusions upon our privacy and liberty. Volunteers are to be warned they are trespassing, and local police are to be called to press charges if they come again after being given a proper trespass notice. (See appendix A) Giving them a legal trespass warning (and a copy of this book) and recording their visit is fair warning. Recordings should be kept for future use so the volunteers can be prosecuted for crimes against humanity at a future date.

It is imperative to win the first round and repulse the invading health volunteers as the warm and fuzzy health ambassadors (aka Blue Assassins) may soon be followed by a not so fuzzy SWAT Strike Team to forcibly vaccinate you or relocate you to a FEMA camp for extermination. If armed intruders enter your home you have the legal and moral right to defend yourself, including deadly force. However, this situation may be resolved by local law enforcement upholding the Constitution and deputizing 100 heavily armed citizens to counter this threat as has done effectively against Black Lives Matter without incident. The paid agitators and rioters were smart enough to get back on their bus and leave. If local law enforcement are reluctant to do their duty then it is up to the citizens to form Committees of Safety as our ancestors did in the Revolutionary War to repel the British troops from incursions into their homes. DO NOT INITIATE ANY VIOLENCE AGAINST THEM. However, having some biker friends duct tape them to a tree would a reasonable response and quite educational as to the errors of their ways. It may possibly save them from being hung by a lamppost like Mussolini later down the road. Treason and Satanism are not to be tolerated. Too bad tar and feathering has gone out of fashion. Appendix A and B have the proper legal forms to notify any agents to leave your property subject to arrest if they return. If the phase 1 blue shirt assassin "health ambassadors" are not stopped cold then it will only lead to phase 2 SWAT TEAMS injecting citizens and hauling them away for torture and death at FEMA camps.

As Mike Adams clearly points out in his Global Reset Survival Guide eBook (www.Brithteon.com) a rural homestead is more defensible against intruders whether they be a Covid Strike Force or Chinese invaders. Having your armed extended family and friends present also affords a more defensible position. Kinfolks are your first line of defense. Gunports in the walls have not been in fashion since the days of Daniel Boone, but I believe they will make a comeback. So will escape tunnels as in the James Bond movie Skyfall.

I also agree that tomahawks, Bowie knives, manchettes, and bayonets are all good for close in work. However before deciding to go all in as in Rambo's Last Blood, I suggest you just leave.

I recommend those who have the means to have an offshore residence in a friendly nation such as Belize or Costa Rica to leave until such time as any possible reign of terror has passed. Communist coups are known for their bloody devastation. Another choice is to have a loaded yacht standing by in Florida for a quick escape to the Bahamas and beyond. Every country in the Caribbean is only a days sail and therefor offers the greatest international protection. Remain a perpetual traveler and sovereign citizen until all dangers have passed. It is essential that the very wealthy leave and remain offshore as if We the People lose this war those with money will be tortured to give their money to the state as in Communist China. This migration offshore has already begun by America's wealthiest citizens. Conversely if a protracted revolution should be started the Constitutional Forces of the Republic will need financing as in the Revolutionary War. Remember George Washington paid his troops with his own money as did the Marquis de Lafayette.

For those on a budget every self-respecting mountain man should have a hunting camp in the mountains or on an inaccessible island and be prepared for the worst. If that is not possible, I encourage you to move to a RED state in a 2nd amendment sanctuary city. At the present time Florida under Governor DeSantis, affords the most Constitutional protection against the disclosure of your health information. Florida has a law making it illegal for anyone to ask about your health status. This was passed as protection against cruise ships demanding to know your health status and requiring the so-called health passports.

The covid controversy will continue and may lead to medical martial law so more people can be killed. It is estimated that half of the vaccinated will die within a couple of years. (Including the useful idiots acting as "health ambassadors".) The plan is to achieve as many vaccinations as possible to reach their quota of 100 million deaths in America. State governors who are aware of this genocidal plan may seek to secede from the union as was done in the first civil war. All of the Southern states and most of the Bible belt states of the Midwest can be expected to secede in response to Federal Communist tyranny. Unless we can stop them at phase 1.

Following Hitler's playbook of the Reichstag fire and 9-11, it is inevitable that there will be some false flag event blamed on anti-vaxxers to discredit them and to promote gun confiscation. I think we will see an Oklahoma City type event with lots of civilians and children killed by gunfire. As before this will be orchestrated by the rogue elements of the FBI and others. Don't be fooled. The use of crisis actors around the world is commonplace. Even the Chinese in Wuhan had citizens dropping dead in the streets on camera. Then they went home for dinner.

However, there are countermeasures beginning with NEVER, EVER, EVER getting a vaccine shot or even a swab. If the bad guys have your DNA, they can target you. We do not want Hitler's New Man. We need enlightened souls with diamond bodies to throw a wrench into the Great Reset. How to do it is outlined in part II of this book.

CHAPTER 9

BRING ON THE LOCKDOWNS

I WAS READING DR. VERNON Coleman's book <u>The Coming Apocalypse</u> about his experiences with Covid-19 in the UK. I really love this guy! He has that great British humor and stiff upper lip. Unlike so many others trying to be so politically correct he expertly summed up our current situation. Dr. Coleman said that "the reaction to Covid-19 has been the biggest cockup in world history or it's a conspiracy. Can politicians really be this stupid?"

Our current crisis began with a covid projection by mathematician Professor Neil Ferguson of the Imperial College of London. His model suggested that 250,000 people would die without social distancing. The case fatality ratios ranges were .5-4.0% and 1.2-5.6. All proved to be too high and actual fatalities that were solely caused by Covid-19 were approximately 8%. Therefore the 73,512 reported deaths in the UK when adjusted for comorbidities were only 5,880. This certainly calls into question the 250,000 projected deaths and is far lower than the usual seasonal flu. We must ask the question as to whether some other more sinister agenda was in play.

An old saying attributed to the Rothschilds is that "the best time to buy is when there is blood in the streets." The financial devastation caused by lockdowns in the UK and the USA and elsewhere creates a buying opportunity for those with cash to buy homes and businesses for a few cents on the dollar. 25% unemployment will take decades to recover. The motto is never let a good crisis go to waste. Draconian police powers granted during a crisis never seem to go away after the crisis has passed. The millions of deaths caused by starvation around the world are a wish fulfilled for the wicked. This may be the worst global recession in history!!

In Bryan Walsh's End time: A Brief Guide to the End of the World, he talks about all the planning that went into the pandemic. There was Event 201 on October 18, 2019, brought to you by the World Economic Forum and Bill Gates as a high-level pandemic EXERCISE that kills 65 million people. Then they tried to refute it. But the planning goes back much further to Operation Dark Winter another senior level bio-terrorist attack simulation by John Hopkins in Jan. 22-23, 2001. They used a smallpox model. The Rockefeller Foundation funded Operation Lockstep. Big surprise. I do not think it is a coincidence that one of the foremost NWO Satanist PREDICTED EXACTLY WHAT HAS HAPPENED DUE TO Covid-19. There is no such thing as coincidence especially since none of the terrible scenarios mention only potential cures or treatment other than their vaccine agenda and or a One World currency. I want to tell you it's all lies as there are both cures and preventions. And a One World currency owned by Satanists is not necessary or desirable. Quite the opposite. We already have a one world currency, and it is called GOLD.

I was reading Covid-19 The Great Reset by Klaus Schwab of the World Economic Forum. (Yeah, I read your book you magnificent bastard!) He says that getting back to a new normal was somehow dependent on good (one world) government and proliferation of a vaccine. Since when have we ever had good government? Haha. I think King Leonidas of Sparta said it best in the movie the 300 when asked to bow down to the king of Persia. "Submission? Now that is going to be a bit of a problem."

The first reason may be the most obvious to some. That being that GOVERNMENT created the virus in the first place as a NWO test run to count the sheep. And to see how many elderlies and "useless eaters" could be killed with it. Making a ton of money was a secondary aim.

Secondly, those who are opposed to the use of untested experimental vaccines for the common good are now ridiculed as "anti-vaxxers." The powers that be will certainly want to make vaccines mandatory with tracking chips to maintain social distancing. This is to prevent a formulation of a revolution as meetings will be needed. (Most of the planning for the American Revolution was done in taverns so of course these were closed.) It has nothing to do with the actual spread of a disease. And if you object to having your child becoming autistic from a vaccine (1/32 chance) then I assure you a second pandemic is planned to get the sheep in line.

Thirdly, practical medical treatments are available and have been used successfully in Taiwan. They use an anti-asthma drug called BUDESONIDE. A country with 25 million people on an island like so many sardines had only 7 deaths. Dr. Richard Bartlett was interviewed on the America Can We Talk TV show with Debbie Georgatos, but apparently the medical establishment missed it. (www.americacanwetalk.org).

Dr. Simone Gold was fired from her job for the sin of curing her Covid-19 patients in 12-48 hours with hydroxychloroquine. Dr. Gold states that over 2 billion does have been prescribed over the counter in other countries by thousands of doctors. The bark of the cinchona tree from Peru has been used for centuries to treat malaria. Even George Washington gave it to his troops to combat malaria. According to Dr. Mercola this is best administered in low doses along with zinc and the antibiotic azithromycin. Although the drug has been considered safe for over 65 years suddenly it is considered unsafe and ineffective. Guess why? It only cost pennies to make, and it works. The tablets cost .60 cents each retail and can be used at home at the earliest onset of a problem. If HCQ had been used in America at least 200,000 lives could have been saved according to Joel S. Hirschhorn in his book **Pandemic Blunder**. But the FDA blocked its use to kill as many as possible. Even the President used HCQ, and this presented the opportunity to villainize the President as well as the drug. And of course, public officials deciding the pandemic response had a financial interest in the costly ($4,000.) and ineffective remdesivir and got their cut. The problem is that if low-cost treatments are readily available and effective there is no need to create a $350 billion-dollar experimental death vaccine and microchip the entire world. Get it? To counter this fraud Dr. Gold has begun a Truth Tour to expose this coverup about treatments and the safety of vaccines. You can watch her here.

https://www.bitchute.com/video/CS{P45qJCJtf/

You can order HCQ online from Dr. Gold's Frontline Doctors and stock up for an emergency. www.americasfrontlinedoctors.com .

Freeze dried crocodile blood will also knock it out in a few days. Its about $160 online (Modaplas Plus). There are 1.2 million crocodiles in Thailand standing by for service. Not surprisingly many farms are owned by the Chinese. The main cause of death from Covid is pneumonia as a secondary infection. Even Fauci admits this. Eventually Western anti-biotics will be useless, and this is an item you can stock up on until you set up a perfected immune system. Earlier vaccines may be full of latent viruses and bacteria including HIV and cancer. I believe Modaplas is strong enough to clear out all latent pathogens. Not only do Covid vaccines carry latent viruses but vaccines going back 70 years are also likely contaminated.

White powdered gold will raise DNA activity to normal within a month even if the subject is near death. Normal DNA activity is 33%. If you have the flu your immunity may be down to 20% or less. White powdered gold will raise immunity by 1% per day. Once you get back to normal keep going. I have been taking it for over a decade. This will help raise your spiritual calibration above the threshold of disease which we will talk about in part II.

At this point you might ask why all the medical establishment, universities, and intelligence agencies around the world with untold trillions of dollars and super- computers at their disposal cannot seem to find a cure for anything? How can an impoverished author find viable treatments and a potential cure in 2 weeks armed only with a laptop on the kitchen table and a cheap cellphone? The first answer is simple. THEY do not give a shit! So, what to do? What are all the anti-vaxxers and patriots going to do? Are there more alternatives? Normally anyone who blows the whistle or cures something and runs afoul of the Nazi agenda find themselves in prison or dead.

The Buddhist would tell you there is always a middle way. In this instance it is a little-known fact that enlightened masters are immune to ALL disease. You have a majority of one. No government in the world can legislate health, but you have the unlimited power of God to create your own. You are the power. God lies within. You are the church. So, if you have given your power away then take it back and be omnipotent. As a man thinketh so he is.

Fortunately, someone foresaw the certain future of a worldwide pandemic and developed a Universal Theory of Disease and Rejuvenation to assist mankind in this troubled time. Lt. Lawrence Frego's **An End to All Disease & the DaVinci Code Revelations** published in 2008, page VII begins with:

"We are at the crossroads of world health. On the one hand we face the possibility of a world-wide pandemic, the likes of which has never been seen before. We are, likewise, on the threshold of discovering natural cures for nearly every disease. As choosing wisely may mean the difference between life and death, this book is designed to help the reader choose alternative options that are seldom if ever in the news."

I have further refined these concepts into a quick and easy **ASCENSION PROTOCOL** and will cover all the supporting material in part II. The reader will question does it really work? The answer is yes. I am on the front lines every day at a hospital emergency room. At another job I saw all 30 of my co-workers get the flu. Everyone was sick as we were outside all winter. Everyone was sick except me!! I healed as many co-workers as I could and healed the damaged lungs of those I could not get to earlier. One extremely sick co-worker was back to work in 2 days with just a 1-hour healing session on her lymph glands and lungs.

My daughter once called me to say she believed she had the bird flu and was dying. I rushed over and healed her for two hours and she was back to school and was a starting volleyball tournament player the next day. Kids do not listen. What can I say?

Therefore, from my personal experience I can tell you all the Covid madness and deaths are all unnecessary. Any experienced Reiki master can heal you in a couple hours unless you have several co-morbidities. Then it will take longer. You can easily learn the ascension protocol and be extremely resistant, if not immune to all disease. Once you complete your lessons treating covid is a piece of cake!!

Old Klaus Schwab of the World Economic Forum says that "No one will be safe until everyone is vaccinated". Well, that's gonna be a problem. (I read your book you magnificent bastard!!) First, who appointed him spokesman for the world? Jacob Rothschild? Klaus Barbie? I would like to know. I have a better idea. How about we have our government quit spraying chemtrails, poisoning our food, and allowing GMOs. Stop all the vaccines full of mercury, aluminum, smart dust and RDIF tracking chips. Cancel 5G.

The truth is no one will be safe until we lock up or eliminate the Satanic 13 families. Why should one small group of pedophiles and murderers have all the world's wealth? Want social programs and a guaranteed income for all the poor. Then let us start with the Rothschild's $500 trillion. That would buy a lot of social justice. Let us put THEM in the death camps THEY made for US. See how they like it. They can all join Marie Antoinette as far as I am concerned.

Informed individuals have some inkling of what Bill Gates and Microsoft are up to in their push to microchip the world and link us all a cyber currency and the Mark of the Beast as predicted in the bible. That is just the tip of the iceberg of the deeper conspiracy. What most people do not know is convicted sex trafficker and rapist Jeffrey Epstein and Bill Gates were very close and working on the same charitable foundations to bring about the great reset. Epstein once confessed to being a CIA agent, but later recanted. However, he also had close contact with the Clinton Foundation and therefore Hillary Clinton, Bill's CIA handler. Bill Clinton as you can expect was a frequent visitor to Epstein's Orgy Island as it is called. No surprise there. However other Microsoft executives were involved with Epstein. Where it gets interesting is that socialite Ghislaine Maxwell was Epstein's girlfriend and allegedly his partner in sex trafficking crimes. She is the daughter of Robert Maxwell, the notorious Israeli spy master. And it appears the whole Maxwell family participated in computer software companies developed by former Israeli Intelligence Officers. Epstein and his girlfriend were high rolling fixers and supplied women for Prince Andrew and the Royal family. A real shocker is that Bill Gates appears to have been dating Ghislaine Maxwell's sister Isabel, despite being married. (Hence his upcoming nasty divorce.) The computer software involved has been used in intelligence linked sexual blackmail operations set up by Jeffrey Epstein. And finally, Epstein science advisor was Melanie Walker a celebrated neurosurgeon. She was "given" to Prince Andrew as a sexual gift. Microsoft and the World Economic Forum are business partners and linked to Isabel Maxwell and the Israeli espionage linked company CommTouch. And some of Epstein's girls are "advisors" to the World Economic Forum. They are all linked to the premier Satanic Black Nobility family via the Rockefeller Foundation. The bottom line is that all the players are on the same white slavery, sex trafficking, drug, blackmail, and espionage team. Yet they are regarded as respectable. They all need to be exposed. To read the whole story go to www.drmercola.com and read: The Truth About Bill Gates, Microsoft and Jeffrey Epstein by Whitney Webb. I am sure you will find it enlightening.

We all need to survive and ascend until the next incarnation of Christ. SHE will be here soon. Until then- kick them down a well.

CHAPTER 10

THE COVID-19 HOAX

ONCE AGAIN FOR THE 10TH time in the last decade we are "On the Eve of Destruction." It appears the first casualty of any new false flag operation is the truth. Plagues are nothing new in history. They happen all the time. What is new are man-made bio-terror weapons deployed to kill the enemy, ruin the enemy's financial markets, and disable resistance to make conquest easier. Unfortunately, We the People are the new enemy. Keep this fact in mind as we go ahead with both the cause and the solution to the global pandemic.

Jared Diamond brilliantly pointed out in Collapse: How Societies Choose to Fail or Succeed that only civilizations that recognize the threats against their existence, and deal with the threat effectively survive. The purpose of this article is to propose effective solutions.

First, we must recognize the fact that we have been down this road before. The expert talking heads of the AIDS pandemic tried to sell us the green monkey theory of origination. I am sure it was just a coincidence that AIDS first appeared near Nazi owned land (missile sites) in Africa. The whistleblowers who revealed that AIDS was a genetically engineered combination of sheep visna virus and bovine leukemia made at Ft. Detrick, MD. soon found themselves dead.

The infected bat theory sold at the Wuhan, China market doesn't have much credibility in light of the fact that it appeared just a few miles from the Wuhan Institute of Virology. Is it another coincidence that doctors (whistleblowers?) from this facility are missing and presumed dead? Another coincidence is that Mr. Du Wei, the Chinese ambassador to Israel also turned up dead. Imagine that! Testing of exceedingly dangerous "chimera" virus was outlawed in the USA in 2014, so the NIH apparently outsourced this testing to China. The bottom line is that your tax money paid for the creation of Covid-19. We can debate whether it escaped or was strategically deployed for political ends. A close examination of the evidence will help you choose wisely. It may not even be a contagious virus at all!!

I rarely pay attention to medical experts as in general they tend to be ethnocentric. I do feel that Dr. Luc Montagnier, the French virologist and winner of the Nobel Prize (2008) in Physiology or Medicine for his discovery of HIV is a credible witness. Dr. Montagnier has said that the "presence of elements of HIV and germ of malaria in the genome of Coronavirus is highly suspect and the characteristics of the virus could not have arisen naturally." (Wikipedia) This is a polite way of saying that HIV, SARS, and MERS could ONLY have combined in a high-level laboratory.

This may be the first time in history that a fraud brought the whole civilized world to a standstill. Conspiracy theories abound on social media. Bloggers want to know who is behind killing grandma and grandpa. And why would our government pay a doctor $39,000 to list a death certificate as COV-19? My favorite headline is "Man shot in the head 33 times dies of COV-19."

Dr. Rashid A. Buttar is the medical director of the Center for Advanced Medicine and Clinical Research in Charlotte, North Carolina and was formerly a Brigade surgeon. His credentials are 3 pages long. (1) He was recently on YouTube telling the public what a hoax the COV-19 pandemic is in no uncertain terms. He says that many government claims are not only fictitious but medically impossible!

Dr. Judy Mikovits, PhD, was previously jailed by Dr. Anthony Fauci of the NIH for her outspoken criticism of vaccine safety and government corruption. She claims that the current pandemic is the intended outcome from the creation of vaccines. You can find her 9-part series on YouTube for details.

I would estimate the actual number of deaths from the virus to be inflated by a factor of 20 xs. It appears that 48% of the deaths occurred in patients nearly 80 years old with a minimum of 3 potentially terminal conditions. 24% had 2 conditions, and 24% had only 1 previous condition. Therefore, I believe what we have seen is the hijacking of "normal" mortality rates into an irrational pandemic. CBS News was caught substituting overcrowded hospital news footage from Italy and passing it off as NYC. They admitted the "mistake" and then did it again in Pennsylvania. My point is the media has blown the whole pandemic out of proportion to the facts and is obviously the mother of all false flag operations. Most recently it was uncovered that the hospital spokesman for Elmhurst Hospital Coleen Smith is a simulation expert. The "Ground Zero" full of bodies had none. Independent researchers around the world have discovered that "expert spokesmen" are nothing more than paid crisis actors and hospital beds are empty, and all the ambulances are in the garage. (https//www.henry makow.com) The Corona Virus is Another Live Drill according to Henry Makow.

Any discussion of the current pandemic would be incomplete without mentioning The Bill and Belinda Gates Foundation and their sudden goal of saving the world with a vaccine. Mr. Gates has a financial interest in several vaccine companies. Therefore, average folks are wondering if he created the whole scenario to make $ billions of dollars or to just kill off millions of "useless eaters" as the NWO calls us. People are concerned that any vaccine that he may develop may have microchips, smart dots or smart dust to tract us and monitor our health. Mr. Gates would like everyone to have a vaccine certificate before going to work. (ID 2020) Therefore many people are accusing Mr.

Gates of being the anti-Christ and the government of Italy wants to have him put into prison for crimes against humanity. Many conservative Christians believe any microchipped device mandated by government is obviously the Mark of the Beast as mentioned in the Book of Revelations. I can only say that my landlord Irving had a number tattooed on his arm. He got it from the Nazis at Treblinka concentration camp in WWII. I am afraid Mr. Gates has embraced the dark side of the force and now has a spiritual calibration only slightly higher than the actual anti-Christ and Hillary Clinton. The truth has many layers like a Russian Matryoshka nesting doll and is indeed stranger than fiction. We must therefore begin to peel away the layers to find it.

The media is busy whipping up the vaccine hysteria. And they keep telling us there are no treatments or cures. Let me translate "med speak" for you. What they really mean is that there is not much THEY can profit from now. Eventually THEY will save us all and only charge us a few $ billion for research and development. And a small percentage may die about equal to those who might have died from the virus. But that is ok. THEY really hate it when you seek alternative treatment of any kind as that ruins profits.

Those of us who are old enough remember when the FDA was trying to outlaw vitamins and make them only available by prescription. They spent millions trying to talk ordinary folks out of taking vitamins. That may be because the latest data shows that vitamin D in sufficient quantities cuts flu mortality by about 50%. Back in 1918 and the days of the Spanish flu there were no anti-biotics. Troop ships would pull into port with hundreds of cases. Thousands of tents were set up by medical staff and the infected troops stayed in their tents at night and were moved into the sunlight during the day. Doctors believed that fresh air and sunshine (vitamin D) reduced mortality by 40%.

Areas in Italy that have groundwater with high selenium content had 3x less mortality. Certain areas in China also have high selenium content.

Apparently, viruses have an Achilles heel. They cannot live in elevated temperatures above 133 degrees. Therefore, time spent in the sauna can kill them all including the common cold which is a great money maker every year. If you do not have access to a sauna very cautious use of a hair dryer will do the job.

Maverick doctors are using Schweppes' tonic water and zinc to relieve symptoms. They say that tonic water has a small amount of quinine in it. Quinine is an anti-malaria drug that has been in use for ages and used to be available over the counter. The President Trump himself says he takes an anti-malarial drug called hydroxychloroquine. When taken in combination with other drugs it seems to be effective.

Andry Rajoelina, the President of Madagascar, states his country has a history of traditional medicine. He claims his compatriots use Covid-Organics and there have been no deaths. Therefore, he urged all African nations to expel the WHO and let them take a hike.

Dr. Richard Bartlett was recently on the Debbie Georgatos show America Can We Talk? (www.americacanwetalk.org) and stated he had achieved a 100% recovery rate using an anti-asthma drug called BUDESONIDE. It is used in an aerosol form and even elderly patients with cancer (the highest risk group) recovered in a few days. He stated that this treatment is used extensively in Taiwan and that although the country has 25 million people packed in like sardines the country has experienced only 7 deaths.

I again mention Dr. Simone Gold of Front-Line Doctors who states that hydroxychloroquine can reverse covid in 12-48 hours. Watch her Truth Tour for all the details. See www.americasfrontlinedoctors.com .

Back in the year 2000 a BBC News team when to Australia to make a documentary on crocodiles. The producer, Jill Fullerton-Smith noticed that crocodiles never became infected despite horrendous injuries incurred. Therefore, she sent samples to be analyzed by a lab in the UK. The lab was able to isolate the active ingredients and a new anti-biotic industry was born in Thailand. The freeze-dried crocodile blood is amazingly effective against all bacteria and viruses including those that are resistant to current anti-biotics.

This was first published on March 17th, 2000 in an article entitled "Croc Blood Battles Superbugs." There are currently an estimated 1.2 million crocodiles on farms in Thailand, many of which are owned by the Chinese. Thailand is the sex tourism capital of the world and had a rampant AIDS pandemic until the introduction of "Crocodillon" as we call it. As freeze-dried crocodile blood may indeed knock out bacteria and viruses associated with AIDS and cancer you NEVER hear about it in the USA. (Although American researchers at Louisiana State University in Baton Rouge have discovered that the American alligator blood also has the same immunity and destroys most HIV.) Bad for business. You can obtain freeze dried crocodile blood from Thailand (Modaplas) for about $160 and it takes 3 weeks for delivery. It has also been proven highly effective for younger looking skin by Thailand University. I tried it myself to be sure it had no side effects. This is in no way a permanent "cure" for disease, but it is handy to keep in reserve in your medicine cabinet just in case. We will discuss more permanent solutions later in this book.

The news media has totally ignored the fact that any experienced Reiki Master can heal the flu in about 2-3 hours and the client can be back to work the next day. I have done this personally. As I have 25 years healing experience and over 1,000s healings done for clients I would estimate a healing time of about 5 minutes. Reiki is the most popular form of healing in the USA with an estimated 1 million Reiki masters initiated. More than enough to go around. So why are there NO stories about Reiki healers in the news? I was looking for a Bible quote about Jesus commanding his disciples to heal the sick. (Luke 10:9) An article by an anonymous cleric (who is a Satanist in disguise) mentioned healing and witchdoctors in the same sentence to mislead the public. And I thought the days of the Spanish inquisition and burning witches were over. Perhaps that is why most hospitals do not allow healers in although admitting Reiki master healers to hospitals is on the rise. But you never hear of success stories. That is because the bad guys control the news, and the medical monopoly cannot profit from it. It is that simple. I would estimate that several 100,000 posts about Reiki healing the flu and

Covid-19 have been deleted to tow the party line. Is it even possible that 1 million Reiki masters have been silent? I don't believe so.

I would like to say unequivocally that none of the above are "cures" for COVID-19. The most any of them can accomplish is a one-shot treatment. Even if we had a practical vaccine nature has its own way around them. Viruses mutate and what works today may not work tomorrow. There are NO permanent and lasting effects and only against one specific virus. Some of the new vaccines on the market are rated at only 65% effectiveness and that may be a huge lie. Apparently, they don't stop transmission at all because the "disease" is not infectious. What is really needed is a more permanent protocol against all disease. We will outline this approach at the end of this book. But first we must look at the big picture and see what is going on behind the curtain. In the final analysis you may be shocked to learn that the conspiracy theorist in the tinfoil hat was correct all along.

The ultimate big hairy question is whether an actual Covid-19 virus exists at all. Western medicine ASSUMES viruses are infectious and promotes vaccines on this assumption. Contrary to this position other medical researchers claim that the body creates viruses as an immune system response and are therefore non-infectious. They claim that it is more proper to label them exomes. Apparently an actual covid-19 virus has never been isolated or proven to exist. Professor Christine Massey researched 40 countries and inquired if anyone had isolated a covid-19 virus. No one had. If you try to pull up her research on Google, the search engine just spins and times out. Her data is being blocked.

If a disease existed, it could be proven by fulfilling Koch's Postulates and could be replicated. Obviously, it is impossible to replicate a disease that does not exist. The germ theory of disease controversy has been an ongoing battle for over 100 years with the con man Louis Pasteur vs Bechamp. Pasteur won the controversy as it was profitable to assume the germ theory of disease.

The pharmaceutical industry profits from 100s of millions of prescriptions and makes $ billions per day. Western civilization could have been spared untold misery if Bechamp had won.

If indeed the man in the tinfoil hat is the one telling the truth we must ask two critical questions:

If there is no such thing as an infectious covid-19 virus, why was the whole world locked down?

What is the true nature of the alleged Covid-19?

The answer to question #1 is quite simple but of biblical significance. The purpose of Covid-19 is to destroy the world economy and usher in the NWO and the Mark of the Beast cashless society. The Chinese have already rolled out the digital Yuan.

I would admit the whole infectious virus theory fooled me for a year and took many 1,000s of pages of reading to figure it out. Now I would define the real nature of Covid-19 as **RADIATION SICKNESS** and that the seasonal flu was hijacked to cover it up. Have you ever accidently placed an aluminum pan in a microwave oven and set it on fire? The secret government has been spraying chemtrails full of aluminum for over 60 years. Vaccines also have aluminum, mercury and other heavy metals. Air pollution has several heavy metals. **When microwave energy hits all the accumulated metals in your lungs a flu-like reaction occurs. The Wuhan pandemic occurred shortly after the city turned on 10,000 microwave 5G towers. And the same holds true for other industrialized cities when 5G was introduced.** The more air pollution that may be present the more severe the symptoms. For example, if you cross reference the cities in Northern Italy that have the most air pollution with the greatest impact of Covid you will see you will see they match.

5G is just below military grade. Several hundred doctors have filed protests to its use due to its known adverse health effects. The NWO plan is to build millions of towers and link them to a million Elon Musk satellites in space. If everyone on Earth can be microchipped via vaccines and linked to a cyber currency, then the entire world is enslaved. That is the goal. If you do not do as you are told, then your funds are cut off and you starve. However, Mother Earth and the sun may have different plans. One good solar flare of 40% of the sun's volume and the satellites connecting the web of control may all come crashing back to Earth.

Enslavement would be bad enough, but the goal of the NWO is a 90% reduction in population by either sterilization or outright exterminations. The US military has developed 100G capacity for crowd control as being irradiated burns the skin. If the population can be induced to having enough aluminum and heavy metals into their bodies via vaccinations (or by chemtrails) it may be possible to kill everyone in 1-2 hours. Or once all the cell towers are built in each area the population can be herded like cattle and driven away from their homes. All that is needed then is a cattle car to deliver the targets to a FEMA extermination camp. Some cattle cars already are fitted with guillotines so they can slice and dice you before you even arrive.

Incredible amounts of subterfuge, propaganda and fake news are needed to induce the population to pay for their own extermination. That's why the fake media tells everyone Covid is contagious 2.3 million times a month. The Covid-19 hoax is the perfect storm as the data is so easy to manipulate. The definition of the virus can be changed at will. The cycles of isolation for testing can be changed at will. Any new rounds of death can be blamed on a mutated strain. There will be round after round of new alleged strains to encourage the younger population to be vaccinated and build up their toxic load. The young must be sterilized the old must be killed.

CHAPTER 11

AND THE BAND PLAYED ON

THE GLOBAL CONSPIRACY TO PROMOTE false panic about Covid-19 has taken several surprising turns all aimed at promoting world government and "cooperation" to protect us. I will first reiterate that NO ONE has isolated an Covid-19 virus nor the alleged Delta variant. Covid does NOT fulfill Koch's Postulates and therefore cannot be proven to even exist more yet contagious. Furthermore, viruses appear to be the body's immune response to toxicity and excessive EMF exposure (like 5G) reacting with aluminum and mercury in the body to produce a **"FLU-LIKE" SYMPTOM**!! The symptoms are distinctly different from the regular season flu, most notably a dry cough. But no one mentions this. And victims don't generally just drop dead walking down the street with the seasonal flu. Quite the distinction.

The bad guys are continuously pushing the infectious pandemic down every orifice of the public in non-stop fear mongering to achieve their globalist aims. Once you realize this you are on solid ground.

An excellent case study of the nefarious global agenda can be found by examining the drama and deaths aboard the Diamond Princess Cruise ship out of Yokohama, Japan in February 2020. Allegedly 691 passengers were "infected" with the corona virus out of 2,666 passengers. 13 deaths were reported, and the ship was therefore quarantined. The obvious question is- if Covid is a hoax- what really killed the passengers and made the others sick? If you watch the video LEARN WHY COVID IS ACTUALLY TOXICITY FROM VACCINES AND EMF EXPOSURE from www.toolsforfreedom.com , you will see the Diamond Princess has an extremely powerful 5G satellite system called MedallionNet. It is not actually Wi-Fi but has a stronger pulsed frequency array. Its huge! Its state-of-the-art military grade. While I am sure it supplies a strong signal for cellphones and video entertainment, the EMF can damage DNA and the heart. The elderly, immune compromised with co-morbidities and toxicity CAN'T withstand 5G and require hospitalizations. Improper treatment such as excessive ventilation can lead to death. I believe this is exactly what happened. There never was, nor will there ever be an infectious agent present. Just a natural immune response to EMF and toxicity. It would further the cause of freedom from this fraud if some attorney brought charges of wrongful death and charges of false imprisonment against the owners of the Diamond Princess. This would give the world an opportunity to present the real cause of the pandemic and perhaps end the scam and the planned holocaust.

The false flag pandemic is again reaching epic proportions in the UK. The new voluntary lockdown called Pingdemic has quarantined 1.73 million Britons due to the alleged Delta Variant Covid. Anyone testing positive (from the false tests) can receive a ping on their cellphone recommending them to self-quarantine for 10 days. This will create massive infrastructure shortages, particularly food and gasoline. This may ultimately lead to the self-created global economic depression that is planned to usher in the global currency.

I don't think you have to be a Mensa member to figure out the gameplan of the wicked, but just in case I will outline it for you. As Donald Trump often said the public is being treated like suckers. Although the fear mongering has already begun with the Delta Variant scam, the normal seasonal flu will be hijacked **AGAIN** as Covid as was done last year. The spike proteins in the so-called vaccines will be carrying SARS, MERS, 1918 flu, bird flu, cancer and HIV to create the epidemic they say they are offering protection from. Therefore, there will be less immunity and millions of deaths. (Estimated at 50 million). The deaths will be blamed on the unvaccinated, although the vaccinated will die at a rate of 8-40x more than the unvaccinated. More 5G towers and satellites will go up broadcasting ever increasing amounts of EMFs. The environment will be impacted. Life on Earth will hang in the balance. The next round of the pandemic will require 3 booster shots to protect you from the Delta Variant and everyone will be infected with more viruses, aluminum, and mercury. The scam will continue until either 100 million Americans are killed or the public refuses to cooperate and begin effective countermeasures ending the global genocidal plot.

Governor DeSantis of Florida seems to be the only one who really gets it. Florida currently has the highest number of cases. This could be a natural occurrence as Florida has a significant elderly population. It is also plausible that chemtrail spraying and 5G strengths are being increased for political purposes as DeSantis may run for president in the event Donald Trump doesn't run. He also outlawed the health passport and has strong anti-riot laws. I am inclined to believe nothing in this world happens by accident. All the bad guys must do to attack a political challenge to their regime is to increase 5G to even higher frequencies in the target areas or state and increase the chemtrail spraying. And the media leads the band that we're having a covid case nightmare and hospitals are full. Which suddenly they are. You can be the judge. If there were a contagious virus then it would burn itself out. So, it will be interesting to see what fiction the bad guys will come up with next in terms of fake science. Lies, damn lies and statistics. And if they get caught in this scam- they'll blame it on the Trump vaccines which were released without testing under project Warp Speed. All very predictable. Just wait and see. Worst of all there will be numerous false flag events blamed on anti-vaxxers with crisis actors to further the gun control agenda.

CHAPTER 12

THE TEN STAGES OF GENOCIDE

THE GENOCIDE EDUCATION PROJECT HTTPS://GENOCIDEED-UCATION.ORG has published the original document developed by Dr. Gregory H. Stanton, a professor at Mary Washington University. Stanton also leads Genocide Watch, a non-profit organization dedicated to the fight against genocide.

The genocidal process starts with prejudice that continues to grow. By knowing the stages of genocide, citizens are better equipped to identify the warning signs and stop the process from continuing. Preventive measures can stop it.

1. CLASSIFICATION:

All cultures have categories to distinguish people into "us and them" by ethnicity, race, religion, or nationality: German and Jew, Hutu and Tutsi. If societies are too segregated (divided) they are most likely to have genocide.

The main way of preventing genocide at this early stage is to develop opportunities in a society for people to work and live together who are from different ethnic, social, national, or religious backgrounds. More tolerance and understanding is needed and the search for common ground.

The battle lines are already being drawn between those who are vaccinated, wearing masks, and perform social distancing and those who are not. They are the "good citizens" who do what they are told to "keep us safe."

2. SYLBOLISM

We give names or other symbols to the classifications of ethnicity, race, religion, or nationality. We name people "Jews" or "gypsies", or distinguish them by colors or dress, and apply them to the members of groups. This is normal, but when hatred is applied everything changes.

Now we have Republicans who need re-education (just like China and Russia), anti-vaxxers, pro-Trump supporters and all are lumped together as white supremacists. Hate is being promoted in a divide and conquer movement to destroy America.

3. DISCRIMINATION

A dominant group (the Deep State) uses law, custom, and political power to deny the rights of other groups. The powerless group may not be given full civil rights or even citizenship.

Unfortunately, the civil rights of almost everyone are being denied in the name of the pandemic. There is no due process or writ of habeous corpus, and anyone can be rounded up and carried off by the Army National Guard for the crime of testing positive on a bogus Covid test. There have been lockdowns all over the world, millions will starve and die. 40 million American's have lost their jobs, and suicide rates are way up. The election was stolen in the USA to bring in more abuse of power and the implementation of vaccine mandates, health passports and a travel pass.

4. DEHUMINAZITION

Dehumanization is when one group treats another group as second-class citizens. Members of a persecuted group may be compared with animals, parasites, insects or diseases. When a group of people is thought of as "less than human" it is easier for the group in control to murder them.

Now we have "super-spreaders", "asymptomatic spreaders" of disease (basically everyone) who are labeled ENEMIES OF THE STATE AND A THREAT TO NATIONAL SECURITY. And doctors who call out the lie of infectious disease are blacklisted and marked for assassination eventually. Even the elderly on Social Security are parasites. They are labeled such as they won't be as missed when the state kills them off.

5. ORGANIZATION

Genocide is always organized, usually by the state, though sometimes informally or by terrorist groups. Special army units or militias are often trained and armed. Plans are made for the genocidal killings.

National Guard units have already been tested to move Covid positive citizens to a treatment facility. Contact tracers are eager to inform on their neighbors and round them up. FEMA continuously drills to respond in national emergencies whether real or imagined. However, they are trained to drive the bus to the camps without thinking about what is happening. As the Nazis all said at Nuremberg, they are just following orders.

6. POLARIZATION

Extremists drive the groups apart. Hate groups broadcast polarizing propaganda. Laws may forbid intermarriage or SOCIAL INTERACTION. Extremist terrorism targets moderates, intimidating and silencing the center.

This is something you see daily on the news. It is all propaganda and censoring. The world is so happy they are being vaccinated. Anyone who is a moderate and recommends a wait and see attitude are vilified as dangerous. Doctors are blacklisted and fired for effectively treating Covid and talking about it. You can be arrested for even mentioning Vitamin C as a possible treatment. Not allowed. Medical licenses are being pulled for the crime of curing Covid with cheap readily available conventional medicines. Every time you try to pull up something on the internet you get a popup with Covid facts and how safe the vaccines are. The good stuff is banned. David Icke's video was banned for instance. Even the President of the USA was banned from Facebook and Twitter and other social media. How insane is that? What happened to freedom of speech? Discussion is not allowed. The powers that be wanting to ram vaccination down everyone's throat and reduce the population. They will use every means necessary to carry out their goals.

Everywhere you look you see polarization and hate groups. The cancel culture. Tearing down statues as they are racist. Does anyone realize this is a classic Communist tactic? Don't Communists tear down Buddhist statues in Tibet? Jihadists also tear down statues in the Middle East. Everyone wants to tear down the past. Why? Because there is no God in Communism. There is no culture except the state.

7. PREPARATIONS

National or perpetrator group leaders plan the "Final Solution" to the Jewish, Armenian, Tutsi or other targeted group "question." They often use euphemisms to cloak their intentions, such as referring to their goals as "ethnic cleansing," "purification", or "counter-terrorism." They build armies, buy weapons, and train their troops and militias. They indoctrinate the populace with fear of the victim group. Leaders often claim, "If we don't kill them, they will kill us."

This is being accomplished daily although the public is totally ignorant and believes that it can't happen here. Well, it already has. FEMA already has 800 death camps ready to go all armed and ready. The lights are on and they are fully manned. The largest one in Alaska is located on 2 million acres and connected by rail to the lower 48. This is destined to be America's Gulag if we let it. It would only take a few months for these camps to liquidate 100 million Americans in the name of stopping the pandemic. The fear of the infected killing the good, vaccinated citizens is a daily occurrence if you are paying attention. This is so they can all be put on the bus and never return. It is estimated that about 40 states governors are onboard the Communist "progressive Democrat" gravy train. Therefore, we are only 3 phone calls away from the new American holocaust. The President calls FEMA to activate, FEMA calls the governors to active the camps. And the camps are called to open the gates. It's that simple. In the event of a rioting scenario Chinese UN troops will be activated to go house to house to round everyone up. So, 4 calls are a possibility. The bottom line is whether the 2nd amendment to the Constitution is intact or not.

8. PERSECUTION

Victims are identified and separated out because of their ethnic or religious identity. Death lists are drawn up. In state sponsored genocide, members of victim groups may be forced to wear identifying symbols. Their property is often confiscated. Sometimes they are even segregated into ghettoes, deported into concentration camps or confined to a famine struck regions and starved. Genocidal massacres begin.

FEMA has already drawn up Red Lists of those to be assassinated during a planned takeover. Artists, intellectuals, prominent citizens, and leaders who oppose the takeover of the country. Not to be outdone Bill Gates thinks DEATH PANELS to decide who is worthy of life and who has "no benefit whatsoever to society" should be created. His idea is to cull the population of the world by 10-15% or about 1 billion. As a Satanist he does not understand that every soul is an expression of God. Or perhaps he does? None of the globalists have volunteered to do their part and kill themselves. They only want to kill us. I guess they are special.

Republicans are already being targeted or purged from the US military. Anti-vaxxers are put into isolation even at West Point. Some are court-martialed. Everyone vaccinated will have an identification mark and a number with all their data. The whole Green Agenda is designed to put low-income workers into a green ghetto where they can be either taken away or killed. All the property of victim groups will be seized as always. Confiscated property will go to the conquering troops for their participation. American land would then grow food to support the Chinese population after all the pesky Americans have been killed and removed.

9. EXTERMINATION

Extermination begins, and quickly becomes the mass killing legally called "genocide." It is "extermination" to the killers because they do not believe their victims to be fully human. When it is sponsored by the state, the armed forces often work with militias to do the killing.

We do not know which groups will be targeted first except for the Red List itself. Bill Gates DEATH PANEL is not specific except to kill all the poor and elderly, particularly in the third world like Africa and India. I believe Africans will be the first major target simply because Africa has lots of gold, diamonds, and oil. The bad guys want all the resources for themselves. Will it be Christians, Jews, Black people, or the unemployed? In Nazi Germany it was systematic beginning with mental hospitals, **the homeless**, and old age homes as these aren't missed. The same protocol may be followed here. That is why homelessness is so encouraged in California with 78,000 building codes. No one misses homeless people.

There are countless ways to exterminate people. Soft kill with toxins, chemtrails, poor medical care, radiation, and the vaccines. Using 100G to irradiate everyone to death is easy. Covert genocide can be carried out by weather modification and starving out a victim country. Its easy to simulate volcanic dust and block out the sun and cause crop failures. Blame it on the weather when everyone starves. This will be the first casualty in Africa as I predict blacks will be the first targets.

And of course, we have the old-fashioned Nazi way with concentration camps, gas chambers, medical experiments, organ harvesting, guillotines, and the ever-faithful firing squad or just buried alive as popular in China.

10. DENIAL

Denial is the tenth stage that always follows genocide. It is among the surest indicators of further genocidal massacres.

Yes, the Deep State will continuously deny any part in mass deaths. Whether it be death by vaccines, starvation, financial collapse, or even earthquakes. They will ALWAYS deny their activity so they can do it repeatedly. The price of freedom is eternal vigilance. All genocidal efforts must be exposed promptly, or they will spread.

FDA DISCLAIMER

The statements made about the effects of the products discussed in this book have not been evaluated by the Food and Drug Administration. Special dietary and nutritional supplements such as these products are intended for special dietary use. They are not intended for use in the treatment, cure, prevention or mitigation of any disease or disorder. They are intended to be used as part of an overall healthy lifestyle program that includes proper diet and exercise. Only your doctor can diagnose and treat any disease of disorder. Before starting to use any nutritional supplement, it is important to check with your doctor.

Second disclaimer: This book is intended for educational and informational purposes only. The author is not a doctor, nor does he claim to be one. The author does not endorse products or websites. The author affirms that he has no financial interest, stock, considerations or received any compensation from any of the companies listed in this book.

CHAPTER ONE

PART II: INTRODUCTION TO THE SOLUTION

IT IS MORE IMPORTANT TO PREVENT THE OCCURANCE OF DISEASE THAN TO SEEK A CURE. CHARAKA- THE FATHER OF AYURVEDA

BENJAMIN FRANKLIN ONCE SAID THAT "an ounce of prevention is worth a pound of cure." Although Franklin was referring to fire prevention at the time, this idiom is just as relevant to disease prevention and immunity today. The first problem is that there are incredible amounts of money to be made MANAGING a disease especially if the treatment can be dragged out profitably for 20-30 years until you die. Therefore, most of Western medicine is focused on managing diseases and trauma care, but prevention is a poor stepchild. To paraphrase Erin Brockovich, "they suck at it." Western medicine is also ethnocentric and rarely looks at ancient cures from other countries, especially herbal or holistic ones as these cannot be patented to make $ billions of dollars. Conversely curing anyone of anything is bad for business!! In America, the FDA stands guardian to ensure natural cures never reach the marketplace or interfere with big pharma and Wall Street investors. If you were to brew a cup of tea and sell it a SWAT Team would soon be at your door. Doctors who develop workable cures for HIV end up in prison. Even authors who expose this corruption end up in prison. Big Pharma offers lucrative second careers for public officials who betray the public's trust. Corruption happens across the board for public servants that will help big business get what they want. Alternative treatments, medicines, herbal remedies are routinely aggressively suppressed as are every other technological advancement that might free the common man. This book is about changing all that and revealing some of the greatest healing secrets you have never heard of.

This part of the book is laid out differently than most. First, I will lay out a condensed version of an innovative approach to Covid-19 specifically and then go ahead to a short version of the ASCENSION PROTOCOL to acquire UNIVERSAL IMMUNITY. Then each aspect of health will be broken down with instructions on how to achieve it. It will take time and some expense to fully implement it and use it, but the results are nothing short of miraculous. Anyone may reprint the protocol providing credit is given to the author. Secondly, we will break down all the steps and discuss common co-factors that need to be addressed for maximum effectiveness. This work is the culmination of 35 years of research and thousands of hours of healing clients with various conditions. I have used these holistic protocols in my own life to great benefit and daily enjoy the fruits of my labors.

If you have already read the chapter entitled THE COVID-19 HOAX, you are already familiar with some of the material we will discuss. To simplify matters let us just say the normal fatalities of the seasonal flu have been hijacked and inflated to cover up the mortalities caused by the weaponized flu. The recovery rate is around 99.97% but is particularly lethal for the elderly and those with 2-3 existing co-morbidities.

To understand why the weaponized flu is fatal for some and not for others we must break it down into its component parts. Apparently, viruses are NOT contagious, but are part of the body's defense mechanism. The body makes viruses (exosomes) in response to attack and acts like a soap to clean dead cells. An immune system that is already overloaded can create too powerful of a response which leads to a cytokine storm. The overloaded system then fails to shut itself back off and thereby can be fatal. 40-50 million of vaccinated people in the USA may die as they discover the hard way the meaning of Antibody Dependent Enhancement Or ADE. Hundreds of millions may die worldwide as they are jabbed with spike proteins. **So, viruses are a response to a toxic environment made by the body. YOU CAN NOT CATCH ONE. So why did everyone wear masks? Why quarantine and social distancing?**

CHAPTER TWO

PHASE ONE OF THE SOLUTION. TAKING OUT THE TRASH.

TO PREVENT OR REVERSE THIS condition we must look at the body terrain. Then we can correct each part of the terrain. This work is the first phase or a pre-treatment to the larger work ahead. To prepare the body for enlightenment you must first take out the garbage.

Using muscle testing I would estimate the components of the weaponized flu-lie symptoms as follows:

47% TOXINS

30% OXYGEN DEFICIENCY

11% VITAMIN AND MINERAL DEFICIENCY

11% EMF RADIATION

1% GENETIC FACTORS

1. **TOXINS.** Toxins are a major factor in all disease in Western civilized society. We live in a toxic world with air, water, and food pollution. Add to this exposure to chemicals, stress, smoking and fungi and bacteria. All of this builds up over the years as a toxic load unless corrective measures are constantly being performed. Truly adverse buildup of toxins can be removed with EDTA chelation. Mystery illness are often the result of mercury AND ALUMINUM as found in many vaccines AND CHEMTRAILS. Dr. Rashid A. Buttar of Charlotte, North Carolina is an expert on toxicity and the author of The 9 Steps to Keep the Doctor Away. Less serious levels of toxicity can be removed with oral chelation which can be obtained without prescription. Your health care provider can perform a hair analysis to detect what level and type of toxicity you may have. Perfect Science Water also has a detox formula and can supply hair analysis for their customers. These formulas are immensely powerful, so a pre-treatment is normally needed. Toxins must be removed slowly as to prevent overloading the body.

A volcanic product called Zeolite may be the best counter-measure for those who have already had a Covid vaccine shot. Liquid Zeolite has a unique, complex crystalline structure. Its honeycomb framework of cavities and channels, like cages, works at the cellular level capturing radioactive particles, heavy metals and toxins and taking them safely out of the body without removing beneficial nutrients. It has been used for over 800 years in Asia and more recently at Chernobyl. I feel it may be the best solution to remove nanoparticles due to its structure.

If you think you are not toxic, take the foot detox challenge. Go to a health spa for a detox or get a home kit for $15.00 or less. You will be surprised how black the pads will be!! Use this before and after Zeolite or Perfect Science Water to test the results. Keep detoxing until you are clear or order a hair analysis. I have an ionic foot detox spa which I obtained for about $150. Keep repeating until you are clear.

Fasting has been practiced for thousands of years to remove toxins. Fasting also lowers blood pressure. Be sure to check with your healthcare provider to be certain you are healthy enough to practice a fast.

Saunas and mineral baths are also excellent. Again, be sure you are physically sound enough to use a sauna and observe all precautions including a spotter or aide (observer).

As we live in a toxic world that pours billions of tons of pollutants in the world annually, it is wise to continuously detoxify and rotate products and methods to be sure you are safe. Detoxifying the pineal gland from fluoride will assist in achieving higher states of consciousness and awareness. Once detoxified you can take Ayurvedic herbs to increase your consciousness and calm your mind. I recommend a herb called Bacopa or Brahmi. Its available at www.toolsforfreedom.com Order # 1029. $26.95.

Colonics also have been used for thousands of years to remove toxic buildups in the colon. Undigested food can form a mass blockage resembling a rubber tire and it stops vitamin and mineral absorption. Massage also helps break up the clogs.

2. **OXYGEN DEFICIENCY**. Proper exercise is necessary for longevity, particularly in the elderly. Oxygen kills germs and bacteria and prevents many conditions. An oxygen meter can be bought at most drugstores or online for about $30. Oxygen supplements are also available online starting at $20-30. I personally use OxyFlow 17. The ancient Indian practice of Pranayama or yoga deep breathing is ideal. The Chinese practice of Tai Chi is especially appropriate for the elderly and helps prevent stagnant energy.

    Difficulty breathing and lack of oxygen are one of the most major symptoms of the regular flu and particularly the weaponized flu. Due to many factors, particularly exposure to radiation, the

bonding angles of oxygen increase to 130 degrees instead of the normal 120 degrees needed for oxygen to bond to hemoglobin. (The interaction with iron is compromised) Therefore, the patient suffocates. Lockdowns and stay at home orders prevent healthy exercise and are counterproductive. The body needs exercise daily.

The riddle of longevity, energy, and bonding angles of oxygen was solved decades ago by a brilliant scientist named Dr. Patrick Flanigan in partnership with Nobel Prize winner Dr. Coanda. Dr. Flanigan's book ELIXIR OF THE AGELESS explains this in detail and I will summarize his finding later in this book. Water is a living crystal charged with energy. (Collapse of the crystalline structure leads to death.) He developed products named Crystal Energy and Megahydrate which I take daily. They correct damaged oxygen bonding angles with continuous use. They cost $45 online. I believe hospital use of these in a saline drip would be amazingly effective and prevent many deaths.

I must add light therapy and put it in the middle between oxygen and vitamins because light does both. Many are aware that **sunlight produces vitamin D** in the body and that vitamin D levels are critical to surviving illness and the flu, both the regular flu and the weaponized version (and the fatal spike protein in the vaccines.) What is lesser known is that the near infrared spectrum of light also **helps the mitochondria cells bond with oxygen and creates cellular energy via ATP.** The result of this process creates an extensive list of benefits. To begin with it lowers inflammation which is a major part of most diseases like heart disease, depression, and cancer. It thins the blood, lowers anxiety, helps wounds heal faster, increases fertility, and lessens wrinkles. In short it improves the body across the board. Most of us however are deficient in sunlight. And the lockdowns didn't help any and only made things worse. I would estimate that the average person needs 6 hours of near infrared photo therapy to close the gap. Many of us work in offices daily and just don't get enough sunlight for optimum health. Near infrared lights are relatively inexpensive at under $100. I bought a larger model for $200 so I could position it over my massage table for clients. The combination of light therapy, massage with castor oil (which regenerates nerves and reduces pain) and Reiki healing is an immensely powerful treatment. However, there are wrap around models that you can fasten around your waist to wear while you're working. Sunlight and fresh air were used extensively to fight the Spanish flu in 1918 and resulted in approximately a 40% increased survival rate. Maintaining optimum light levels is a very proactive way to combat ageing and increase fertility. This is especially relevant as the elderly and fertile young women are the main targets of the Vaccine Death Cult. As there are so many benefits to this therapy, I highly recommend reading **The Ultimate Guide to Red Light Therapy** by Ari Whitten. And enjoy the beach!

3. **VITAMINS AND MINERALS**. Dr. Joel Wallach, N. D. the author of **Dead Doctors Don't Lie**, has stated that lack of vitamins, nitrogen and minerals is the ultimate cause of all deaths. Although the findings are preliminary, what we do know of the survival rates of flu patients in Northern Italy, areas where the drinking water has a high selenium content patients have a 50% reduction in fatalities. Vitamins D and E also have significant effects.

   Before the invention of antibiotics soldiers with the 1918 Spanish flu were treated with fresh air and sunshine. (Vitamin D). they were placed in tents and then put outside during the day. Their increased survival rate was estimated to be 40%.

   Swiss doctors have developed a vitamin protocol called MATH. Inclusion of vitamins C, D, B vitamins and zinc supply protection against the flu. Of those who had the proper level of vitamin D only 5.6% tested positive. See covid19criticalcare.com for the latest updates on treatment and prevention.

   Lastly, mainstream science is unaware of all existing classifications of minerals. The use of Ormus or M-State minerals may revolutionize our understanding of disease. I would estimate normal DNA activity at 33%. The use of white powdered gold increases DNA activity approximately 1% per day. Therefore, even if a patient is near death consumption of white powdered gold may restore normal functioning and immunity in a month. The cost is a mere $45. I have been taking it for over a decade and estimate my immunity to be 1,000 times stronger than an average person.

4. **RADIATION** The last item on our weaponized flu list is EMF radiation, especially 5G. 5G is just below weapons grade. Excessive radiation when combined with toxicity, like chemtrails destroys cellular functioning and oxygen bonding angles. Radiation meters are readily available for use in the home, work or in your car. EMF cancelling devices are available for the home starting at $45. Protective clothing, bracelets, blankets, hats, bed covers, and even a Mombasa style netting for your bed are imbedded with silver fibers. There is a wide range of protective clothing from business suits to maternity dresses. And Faraday boxer briefs. http://getlambs.com. As EMF is a complex subject, we will include a whole chapter on it later in the book. For a better understanding of the subject read Dr. Joseph Mercola's **EMF*D: 5G, Wi-Fi & Cell Phones: Hidden Harms and how to Protect Yourself.**

A patient with the flu or weaponized flu can be stabilized with energy healing such as Japanese Reiki. An experienced Reiki Master can heal all a client's lymph glands in one session, and they are symptom free in 1-2 days and can return to work. Those clients who have damaged lungs due to the flu can quickly be returned to normal breathing and health. I have personally conducted this several times. It is extremely easy to do. Covid symptoms are primarily signs of an energy imbalance in the aura. The symptoms are even more severe in the vaccinated as some vaccinated individuals are magnetic. I believe all mention of using healing to reverse the weaponized flu have been deleted from social media.

If the public at large were aware that EMF radiation (in combination with aluminum from vaccines and chemtrails) causes flu-like symptoms, then it would be more difficult to sell vaccines and microchip the population. Again, I do not believe it is a coincidence that 10,000 5G cell phone towers were activated in Wuhan, China prior to the alleged Covid-19 pandemic. I believe it is all a false flag operation that has been in the planning for 2 decades.

Any discussion of fatalities from the flu would be incomplete without mentioning co-morbidities. We have been told that most fatalities are in patients over 80 years of age with 2-3 comorbidities. The flu is just the last straw that pushed them over the edge. Obesity is the biggest cofactor at 73% of fatalities. Heart disease, cancer, diabetes and high blood pressure are the most frequently mentioned. When we add the 4 previously mentioned co-factors, what we are really seeing is 6-8 comorbidities. If is therefore no surprise that the outcome is often fatal.

The last four comorbidities are reflective of poor diet and the resultant loss of energy. For example, Dr. Bruce West proved that heart disease was preventable with enough vitamin B and niacin. Diets that are too acidic lead to cancer. An alkaline forming diet is recommended. We will discuss food and energy in greater detail in the ensuing chapters.

I am not inventing anything new here at all. Just a reminder that civilization has its hazards for those who have lost touch with the natural world. Yoga masters have been drinking the white milky water of the Ganges for centuries. They have done deep breathing exercises daily. They grow their own food in their bare feet. They cook their food over open fires. And they are aware of the properties of gems and stones. And healing is a way of life for masters and students alike for thousands of years. This is a time to reexamine your life and activities and to bring yourself more in line with the cosmic plan and nature as God intended it to be.

A great deal of propaganda is being spilled daily and appeals to the ignorant masses to get vaccinated. The lies about Covid are broadcast on social media 2.3 million times per month. I saw one yesterday that said, "Man dying of Covid lasts request is that his family be vaccinated." Don't buy into panic porn. However, what is happening is that the vaccinated are having some strange side effects including being magnetized. Wow. And of course, lots of folks simply drop dead. Guess that proves the vaccine is working! **SOME UNVACCINATED PEOPLE ARE REPORTING ILL SIDE EFFECTS AFTER BEING IN CLOSE CONTACK WITH COVID-19 VACCINATED INDIVIDUALS.** These include massive headaches, micro-clots and sudden bruising throughout the body, exceptionally heavy menstrual cycles, among both the young and post-menopausal women, miscarriages, reduction in breast milk, sterility among both women and men, and lastly household pets dying shortly after the owners get the jab.

The good news is that there is a possible inexpensive antidote for Spike Protein Transmission. Pine Needle tincture is a source of suramin which helps you prevent blood clots and protects both your DNA and RNA by preventing unwanted replication. It costs $22.00 order # 9923 at: wwwtoolsforfreedom.com.

The completed Ascension Protocol which we will discuss shortly will supply a very robust immunity for most people and has the potential to greatly expand longevity. As we have discussed in part one, chapter 8 (vaccines) the vaccinated have numerous injected viruses and contaminated cell lines from monkeys, dogs, pigs, cows, and the infamous Wuhan bats. As vaccinations and contaminated cell lines have been around for 70 years the list of latent viruses can be quite long. Latent cancer, HIV, leukemia, MS, Epstein Barr, hepatitis all may reside in your your blood already just waiting like stealth bombs for an opportunity to manifest. Vaccinations lower overall immunity. I am sure the wicked will constantly experiment with the mix of the vaccines to target specific races and to make them more lethal and covert. The variant game will be played until WE THE PEOPLE either put an end to it or everyone is dead. Whichever comes first. And somehow the unvaccinated will be blamed for the variants. Since when can healthy people infect others? George Orwell's 1984 has finally arrived. Up is down, black is white. I believe the ascension protocol will counter all the latent viruses and diseases contained in the vaccines.

Detoxification is critical to removing all the heavy metals from the vaccines and provide greater resistance. White powdered gold may correct DNA damaged by vaccines and promote healthy DNA activity and electrical connectivity. A great deal more research will need to be done to formulate more effective ormus countermeasures.

Blood disorders of all kinds may be the final killers latent in the vaccines. Specifically micro blood clots may kill 50-100 million Americans WITHIN 1-3 YEARS. Therefore, particular attention must be paid to cardio-vascular health and diet with ample vitamins and minerals. While this is indeed scary stuff, it is a also an opportunity to spice up your cooking with herbs and spices that have been around for centuries and are proven to break up blood clots. The following herbs and spices can be added to the diet as a preventive measure: turmeric, ginger, cayenne pepper, vitamin E, garlic, Cassia cinnamon, ginkgo biloba, grape seed extract, dong quai (female ginseng) feverfew, bromelain (from pineapples) almonds, saffron oil, sunflower oil, sunflower seeds, wheat germ oil, and whole grains. **The Complete Book of Ayurvedic Home Remedies** has some excellent recipes for healing teas for the cold and flu. According to Ayurveda medicine colds and flus are the result of inharmonious eating habits. Few Americans are aware that there are 3 body types, and each diet must be in harmony with the 4 seasons. **Ayurveda Cooking for Beginners** provides practical advice and recipes.

Prevention is an incredibly positive approach, however if you do suspect blood clots see your doctor immediately. Some individuals are very genetically susceptible, and complications can lead to death or amputation of limbs. One unfortunate nurse lost both legs and both hands due to being vaccinated, so be vigilant and seek medical treatment if you have any complications.

Never in the history of the world has the population been attacked by experimental bio-warfare agents and spike proteins to depopulate or subjugate the Earth. Honestly, we don't know how effective counter measures such as azomite, chelation, fasting and Perfect Science water will be in removing poisons, nanoparticles, and hydrogel. My gut feeling is that a 10 day fast to purify the blood will have satisfactory results along with other detoxification methods. As they say in The Marines, we must improvise, adapt, and survive. The fate of humanity is at stake.

CHAPTER THREE

PHASE 2 OF THE SOLUTION: THE ASCENSION PROTOCOL.

THE KEY TO THE COSMIC leap of understanding was given to us many years ago by Reiki Master Mokichi Okada (1882-1955) of the Johrei Fellowship. "Okada taught that the cause of humankind's three great miseries sickness, poverty and conflict are spiritual in nature. He referred to them as "spiritual clouds." (3) Disease is therefore spiritual in nature. Mechanical means cannot solve a spiritual problem. All the inventions of man and all the vaccines do not change the original spiritual problem. Only ascension to a higher state of spiritual awareness can.

I began investigating the nature of disease back in 1989 as I felt a cure for the AIDS pandemic and cancer were desperately needed. After surveying 5,000 books I discovered one written by a Reiki master and I immediately KNEW this was my path to healing my broken body. Although I had knocked out all 33 discs of my spine in an auto accident after 3 reiki treatments, I climbed the Andes in Bolivia with a pack. The following year I took my Reiki 1 initiation.

Originally, I was looking for natural cures for AIDS and cancer and had planned to author a book detailing them. The universe had other plans. Books that I did not order arrived and gave me the keys to preventing and healing all diseases.

So, let us begin our cosmic leap with the greatest healing secret known to man and one you have never heard about. Are you ready to think outside the box? How about throwing the box away entirely?

What is disease? How we define it dictates how we approach it. I would begin by defining disease as a syndrome characterized by low frequency vibrations and lack of cellular structure in the body.

Any discussion of the frequencies of disease must begin with the pioneering work of Royal Rife. He proved that every disease has a specific frequency and can be eliminated by an equal and opposite frequency. All diseases begin in the lower frequency bands and health lies in the upper frequency bands. To illustrate this, the major frequency ranges are below:

25 MHz Death begins

42 MHz Cancer

52 MHz Epstein Barr diseases

57 MHz the Flu

58 MHz Colds

62 MHz Normal vibratory rate, lower

68 MHz Normal vibratory rate, upper

72 MHz Optimal brain functioning, lower

75 MHz, Threshold of disease (theoretical)

90 MHz Optimal brain functioning, Upper.

90 MHz threshold of immortality (theoretical)

This information is essential for two reasons. **The first being all that is required to <u>SOFT KILL</u> anyone without them suspecting it is to gradually lower their frequency by radiations such as tv, cell phones, towers, FLOURIDE, canned foods, frozen foods, dead water, and thousands of additives, <u>chemtrails, vaccines,</u> chemicals, and poisons. Secondly the way to regain health and create immunity to all disease is to raise the body frequency above the threshold of disease AND DETOXIFY. It is that simple.**

As the frequency of the body is the key to all health or disease obtaining a reading is highly desirable. You may have several weaknesses in your system that you are totally unaware of. A convenient method is Bioelectromagnetic Response Technology. The BioTracker tests 30 systems in the body by reading the electromagnetic signature of each and can access 35,000 bits of information. This allows the practitioner to access a patients overall health and make recommendations. The cost is relatively inexpensive. See (https://www.circleofhealth.com/biotracker/ . I consider this to be Star Trek technology available today. For an appointment call (860) 384-1527. If every hospital had one it would be a gigantic step forward in preventive medicine.

The spiritual cloud we discussed earlier shows itself first in the body's aura. Fortunately, it is easy to remove. In India there have been fire temples with a continuously lit fire for over 5,000 years. All one must do is sit by a small fire and let your aura pass through the fire and burn off your disease potential. The average person needs about 40 hours of **fire yoga** to be cleansed. Any additional hours above this amount indicate immune system compromise. If you need 50-60 hours of fire yoga this would show your immune system is only operating at 50% effectiveness and you are very susceptible to colds and flu and other opportunistic diseases. As your disease potential is removed toxins come out. Therefore, NEVER DO MORE THAN 2 HOURS OF FIRE YOGA AT A TIME. If you do too many hours you will get sick due to a healing reaction. If you do your fire yoga in the backyard fire pit, please follow the Indian tradition of giving an offering of flowers, salt, butter or sugar to the fire in appreciation for its work. Always show appreciation in your meditations. You can calculate how many hours you need by simple muscle testing.

Buddhists describe the Path to Enlightenment as the only true and valid healing method. There are 3 basic ways to raise your body's frequency above the threshold of disease and onwards towards enlightenment and a Christ level of being. The first method is healing. The second is ingestion of Ormus minerals such as white powdered gold. The third is wearing certain gems and stones for specific healing frequencies. Once you reach enlightenment you will NEVER be sick again as you become resistant to all diseases of the world. Getting there isn't as difficult as you might think. If you start now, you could reach it before the next flu season.

To make any ascension system work we need some sort of measurement system. It is impractical to carry around an electron microscope or some type of cellular voltage meter. A quick and convenient method is needed. I use the behavioral kinesiology or muscle testing system developed by David Hawkins in 2002 and published in his book Power Vs Force. The system is based on a scale of 0-1,000 (Christ level). I personally use an extended version of this developed by Taoist Master Jasmaheen in Australia. You can find these charts in the book: An End to All Disease & the DaVinci Code Revelations. (4)

200 &below	Negative emotions of anger, fear, guilt, or shame.
200	Beginning energy of truth and integrity.
310	Calibration for hope and optimism.
400	Reason and wisdom.
500	Energy of love.
540	Energy of joy.
635	Establishment of a Disease-Free Existence
637	Ageing Free System begins.
668	Food free and able to live on prana.
777	Fluid free existence.
909	Physical Immortality.
1367	Dematerialization and rematerialization.
1450	Ability to Perform "Classic Miracles."

The average person has a spiritual calibration of around 205. However, the threshold of disease does not begin until 635. Therefore, the average person is susceptible to disease as all diseases are in the lower frequency range and spiritual calibration range. Enlightenment begins around 700 and a Christ level of being at 999 and above. The ability to perform "Classic miracles" begins at 1450 on the extended chart. It is possible to go from a medically terminal patient to a miracle worker in a couple of years. As God is unlimited so healing is unlimited. It is possible to go 100,000 degrees ABOVE the Christ level and achieve the diamond body of the saints. All you must do is apply yourself and the secrets of healing.

There are many, many forms of healing in use in the world today. I will use Reiki for our discussion as there are 1 million Reiki masters in the USA and therefore it is the most accessible, easiest to learn and the most cost effective. I believe it is similar to the ancient Indian systems, but the symbols used are in Japanese instead of Sanskrit. Reiki means "universal life force energy" and was received by Master Dr. Mikaomi Usui around March of 1923 on Mt. Kurama. This sacred mountain is in Kyoto, Japan. An ancient Buddhist temple built in the year 770 remains on the mountain.

Reiki is divided into 3 basic levels. Each level raises the spiritual calibration of the initiate by about 100 points. Therefore, the latest values of reiki are as follows: Reiki 1= 312, reiki 2= 410, reiki 3= 540. As we need to get closer to the threshold of disease, I recommend the advanced courses of reiki fire to reach a level of 632 and then Tibetan reiki at 650. All these courses are taught at the International Reiki Training Center by Master William Lee Rand. Reiki training is available throughout the world by certified instructors. (www.reiki.org). I highly recommend this training for all front-line health care workers to protect themselves and their patients. Those of you who have compromised immune systems can heal your lymph glands first and your immunity will bounce back to normal. This is how I heal medical personnel, so they are safe. Think of it as just recharging a battery.

Healing can be incredibly effective in a brief period of time. I have personally healed cases of terminal brain cancer, breast cancer, brain injuries, auto accidents, 33 damaged discs, strokes, flu, food poisoning, blood poising, hepatitis C, mastectomies, cracked ribs, hearing loss, kidney failure, broken chakras and the mother of all disease: STRESS. (My most interesting case was that of a past life serial killer who raped and murdered 300 plus Saracen women during the crusades.)

The average person in the USA needs about 12 hours of targeted healing to their major organs and over 1,000 hours of cellular healing. They just are not aware of it. A buildup of between 500-1,000 hours of targeted reiki healing in any one organ is generally fatal. It can also be fixed quite easily by chakra repair, recharging the immune system, and removing all spiritual blocks. See Barbara Brennan's excellent book, Hands of Light for graphic illustrations of this process.

You may think it is impossible to do thousands of hours of healing. It is simple really. Healing is a way of life. When you watch TV on the couch put your one hand on your head and the other on your heart. When you sleep wrap your hands across yourself like a mummy. You can carry out a hundred hours per day if you do it consistently. Once you reach a certain level your healing ability can double unexpectedly, even weekly. Mine has doubled 4 times this month. The more healing energy you have the less time it takes. Ever think about turning water into wine? All it takes is energy.

The "stealth" damage done to the population of the USA is immense. Extreme stress damages chakras, particularly the base chakra which is the chakra of survival. I would estimate 100 million people now have damaged chakras due to the COVID-19 scare and the financial fallout. Any chakra tear over 12% can be fatal. Think of it as having all your energy drain out. Then the immune system collapses making the body vulnerable to any disease that comes by. I would also estimate that 11 million people in the USA now have chakra damage over 12% and 20 plus years down the line there will be a massive death toll which medical science has no clue. This is a planned event by the forces of darkness who feed off fear and negativity. Chakras can be repaired in a few minutes by a trained master healer. It only takes a few minutes and is as easy as rewinding a clock.

The third level of the new paradigm is alchemy. You may think of this as a fairy tale of ancient chemists who used to try to turn lead into gold. However, the history of alchemy goes back to ancient Egypt where the high priests filled entire rooms full of white powdered gold. It took over $10 million in research to bring back alchemy into the public domain by Arizona farmer David Hudson. He holds the patents on the process and has named the elements Ormus. An ormus element has one less electron than the regular counterparts. There are Ormus elements of gold, platinum, silver, Iridium and rhodium to name a few. They are essential to life and you would die without them in a few seconds. The brain is composed of at least 5% iridium and rhodium. Ormus gold particles increase brain connectivity by 10,000%. Ormus elements are discussed in great length in **An End to All Disease and the DaVinci Code Revelations**, so I will only mention a few points specific to this article. As these elements are unknown to mainstream science, we do not know how much of each element we need for perfect health. Nor do we know which deficiency of them causes which disease. Solving this lack of knowledge will probably wipe out all the major degenerative diseases we know of today. As we do not know how much we need of each element or what frequency we need I suggest cycling through them all and observe the benefits of each. At the same time, we can reinforce our ascension protocol by gradually increasing our body frequency. A brief description follows:

Liquid Chi	Spiritual calibration 443
Vulcan's Treasure	Spiritual calibration 471
Hermes' Elixer	Spiritual calibration 491
Manna Tonic	Spiritual calibration 521

These products are available at www.liquidchi.com. You may wish to calibrate others as well. Just be sure you have the real thing. Even white powdered gold is available for $44.95. White powdered gold increases DNA activity 1% per day. Normal DNA activity is around 33%, but those who are near death may be reduced to only 1-2 %. Therefore, taking white powdered gold can be used to return to normal DNA activity in about a month. Immunity will also return to normal. White powdered gold can be used as either a preventative or an effective treatment for those who are ill with Covid. Continued use of white powdered gold can create an immune system 1000x times stronger than the average. I have been taking it for over a decade.

Gems and stones are used in India to remove negative karma and to increase spiritual calibration. I use man-made diamonds from www.stauer.com as my main tool for removing negative karma. Wearing a 50-carat necklace will generally remove 1,000 points (or samskaras) of negative energy per day. The average person has 180,000 units of negative karma. Wearing diamonds for at least 2 hours per day will get the job done. **I also discovered that approximately 30% of diseases or conditions are karmic**. For example, a recent client had a 5,000% stroke potential. After removal of her negative karma the potential went to almost 0. After 3 healing sessions it was 0. I would calibrate man-made diamonds at around 700 in spiritual calibration; therefore, you can wear them to keep your frequency at a level of enlightenment until you get there. For an in depth look at using gemstones for healing I recommend Krista Mitchell's excellent book entitled: Crystal Reiki.

Once you have achieved enlightenment you may wish to continue use of white powdered gold or wear a necklace of moldavite. Moldavite is a meteorite and is not found naturally on Earth. Therefore, it is a bit expensive ($200.) and rare. It calibrates at 1,250 or the mid-level Christ range. I used one in the shape of a dove which symbolized the Christ energy and had excellent results.

You may also use essential oils in your home as their frequency is extremely high. For example, essence of a rose has a frequency of 320 MHz Idaho blue spruce has a frequency of 600 MHz and above. This may be of use in countering the negative frequencies in the home and help raising your calibration to a higher level. A beginner's kit with 10 oils is available for $40.00.

Once you have completed every task on this list don't make the mistake of thinking you are now Superman and Superwoman. All the rules of a healthy lifestyle still apply. Sorry, but drinking, smoking and whoring are still a no no. The wages of sin remain. Why would you build a house in the morning and tear it down in the evening? Would not make much sense, would it? You MUST pay attention to all the co-factors of health like exercise, diet, organic foods, and toxin removal. I use Km Matol and Perfect Science waters. And always remember you must ascend SLOWLY.

Now that I have covered some of the most ancient techniques for disease "resistance" and health I have a few concluding thoughts. There is an old anti-Vietnam War slogan which states, "Suppose they gave a war, and nobody came?" Let's update that concept and say, "suppose they gave a pandemic, and no one got sick." There will be a phase two of this pandemic as surely as the sun comes up in the morning. Hopefully, it won't be for another 10 years as suggested by psychic Sylvia Browne, and we have some time. However, every year there will be something!! If millions and millions of people use the ascension protocol and become "resistant" to all disease, then it would throw a major wrench into the hopes of the wicked. I'd say that millions of enlightened masters would give the NWO "masters of the universe" night sweats. It would be harder to get everyone on the bus to the camps if no one was ill. However, if you don't heed my advice then heads will roll. Death is a grave mistake. It's up to you to decide.

Light ALWAYS triumphs over darkness. Whether it is a long hard road or a shorter one depends on the spiritual evolution of humanity. The more people that are evolved the easier it will be for all. The all-out efforts by the powers of darkness to control the world makes about as much sense as fleas fighting over who owns the dog. Mother Earth has her own plans for population control. If you look at the projections for the future, you may find your state or county isn't there. In the I AM America Atlas it appears that half the current world is going to be underwater. As the Earth's core is heating up, we can expect a higher sea level and some big 100 foot plus tsunamis in the future. I would say in the next 5 years. And the sun is projected to throw out some massive solar flares like the world has never seen before. Possible life extinction events. Increasing your spiritual calibration and psychic potential may keep you out of harm's way. I plan to buy oceanfront property in East Tennessee when the time comes. We may have another 80 years before the ascension of the planet itself and the universe into the 4th dimension. My advice is to go with the cosmic flow and ascend gracefully and enjoy the ride. To paraphrase Mr. Gandhi, I believe the 2,000 Satanists cannot control 328 million Americans if we Americans refuse to cooperate! Do not get on the bus!

CHAPTER FOUR

SECRETS OF HEALING

WE HAVE MENTIONED REIKI MASTER Mokichi Okada of the Johrei Fellowship and his belief in "spiritual clouds" as the cause of all of humanity's problems. These spiritual clouds can be broken down into 5 major categories and then be removed.

In the Siddha yoga tradition going back tens of thousands of years the 5 major blocks are as follows:

1. Birth trauma

2. Parental disapproval syndrome

3. Specific negatives

4. Unconscious death urge

5. Negative karma

Sondra Ray is a student of the 1,700-year-old master known simply as Babaji. She brought the Siddha tradition back to America in the 1970s to Haight Ashbury, San Francisco with Leonard Orr. This tradition employs rebirthing to get to the heart of one's inner trauma. Sondra and Marcus

Ray documented the process in their book entitled: <u>Liberation Breathing</u>. Guided rebirthing can be done remotely via Skype with Sondra and Marcus for a small fee.

Teal Swan was imprisoned by a cult member for 13 years. She developed a process to heal trauma she called the Completion Process. Her experiences and her system are described in her book **The Completion: The Practice of Putting Yourself Back Together Again.** She offers online seminars and has a wellness center in Costa Rica. See http://tealswan.com for more details. I found her protocols to be extremely helpful in understanding how trauma affects behavior and how to remove it.

Negative karma removal has already been discussed using gems and stones. Fire yoga is also of great benefit.

Death potential can be removed with just a hug or a kiss from a master or guru. A more in-depth method I call the yoga kiss which is an alternating breath exchange between the healer and the student. Sitting in the tantric yab yum position (fully clothed) the inner cosmic orbit of the recipient can also be restored. The connection to God is then healed. The only catch is only a small portion of death potential can be removed at one time as the master absorbs the negative energy and must only remove a safe amount. I have made that mistake before and nearly passed out. Babaji showed me how to do this but as usual I was too gung-ho.

Unless the underlying negativity is removed healing is just a waste of the masters' time. An individual with an extraordinarily strong death wishes or unconscious death urge will just seek new ways to kill themselves. All guilt and negativity must be removed, or it will just be a never-ending drama like a country song. If it were not for bad luck, he/she would have no luck at all. Remember however that all souls have free will. If the subject chooses to die, then it is their right to do so. Do not try to force someone to live if they do not want to. They may have other plans and other destinies. That is between them and God.

I had one client who was an extreme alcoholic. He begged me to heal him as he was literally dying. So, I took him in and healed him for many months. After about 25 hours of healing, he was in perfect condition, clean and sober, taking vitamins, working out and even his hepatitis C vanished. (To the great surprise of his doctor.) Then he tried to kill himself with 2 bottles of Kentucky Gentleman whiskey.

Another client had quite the run of "bad luck" as they call it. Breast cancer, mastectomy, hit by a car while jogging, set another car on fire and was nearly murdered several times. My analysis was that she was something of a serial killer in a past life raping and murdering over 300 Saracen women during the crusades. I could see about 80 malicious entities attached to her which were probably those of women she had murdered in that life. What I saw was like opening Pandora's Box. Very scary. I taught her to use the power of Christ to remove them. We also did 300 plus hours of healing as she had been a prostitute in this life. We also did the yoga kiss weekly to keep her out of trouble and to avoid being killed. I could see her in the morgue with students dissecting her and laughing. Whenever she was approaching a dangerous situation from muggers to deer on the highway, I would text her and suggest she make other plans. I learned a great deal from her as Babaji showed me in my sleep how to heal her chakras, remove death potential and keep her safe. She retired from the oldest profession and got married. It took a tremendous amount of work.

It can be a real surprise what is holding you back from your true God potential. A dear friend was having heart problems, so I loaned her a 50-carat diamond necklace from www.Stauer.com and we did some healing. I esti-mated her stroke potential at 5,000%. Once her karma was cleared it vanished. We also discovered a past life bullet hole from WWI. When I ran my hand over her upper chest and felt a sudden draw of energy she got ZAPPED and sat up on the table out of breath. After finding a few more bullet holes she was cleared.

I found a great t-shirt store at the mall. It says, **"You have to let that shit go- Buddha."** I sometimes wear it when healing clients.

Previously I mentioned an 85-year-old college disc jockey I met while studying the Hindu bible. I like to peek inside of the people I meet and see their spiritual calibration and how many hours of healing they may need. I was surprised at this gentleman as his spiritual calibration was so high and he needed no healing from me at all. I asked him how he did it and he told me he lived in an ashram in Spain for 13 years and his guru taught him how to heal. That was his secret.

The universe is in perfect harmony, but at times we are out of balance with it and hence out of balance with ourselves. At such times we need healing to regain our inherent harmonious state.

Contrary to the opinion of some, healing did not stop occurring 2,000 years ago. It has always been present as a gift to those who serve others. ANYONE can learn to become a healer. It is only a matter of intent and dedication. And the purer a channel of love you are, the more power to heal you will receive. It takes only three weekends to learn to become a Reiki healer and receive it's blessing to you for the rest of your life. There are over 1 million reiki master in the USA. The most well known is The International Center for Reiki Training with master William Lee Rand www.reiki.org.

I began with Japanese Reiki in the tradition of Dr. Usui (1865-1926) and within the first hour of instruction I was able to heal others. (Our textbook was Essential Reiki by Diane Stein.) When I was initiated into the second degree of Reiki it felt as though a bolt of lightning hit me in the head. It felt like a spark four inches long. I was so charged up, my hands kept me awake at night. Eventually I completed level III and after daily treatment upon myself I was again able to live a normal life instead of the years of pain I had endured previously due to several car accidents and 33 damaged discs in my back. Reiki saved my life.

There are many amazing things about Reiki energy. It seems to have a mind of its own and heals the weakest link first. I took Reiki with the hope of healing my damaged neck and back. Indeed, discs did jump back into place on their own. But my hearing also improved 100% within the first 15 minutes of treatment. And internal organs such as kidneys and such heated up like hot coals burning out of my body and then completely healed also. I had no idea anything else was even wrong. Having learned this lesson, I spent a year working on each section of my body, sometimes for a couple of hours per day. I regained the strength in my arms and legs. And adverse energy passed out of my feet like gout exiting my body. Reiki also seems to increase fertility dramatically so be prepared.

When I treat others, I see the energy patterns of illness just like an X-ray or simply feel it. Sometimes I see a past life situation or a genetic memory. I was lying in bed one day doing Reiki when I felt an incredible pain go through my left thigh. I could "see" a past life lance going through my leg. In my case the lance had been a real lance, thrown by someone in the Trojan War, I felt, as I viewed the battle. I lost this battle as I was first hit with the lance in the leg and then arrows and swords everywhere. The pain in the leg was excruciating. (In the present tense) until it heated up with healing energy and passed safely out my foot. Quite an experience and the slide show of the battle was fascinating. My leg was stronger after this past life lance had been removed by Reiki healing. Depictions of past life lances are to be found in Barbara Brennan's excellent volume <u>Hands of Light</u>.

Reiki can be immensely powerful and heal the seemingly impossible. My Reiki master told us a story about her sensei who was run over by a logging truck while driving her VW beetle. Her car was crushed flat like a pancake, her ribs and hips were broken. She was torn up quite badly and was in a coma for 3 days. Her students all came and performed a Reiki marathon with dozens of people treating her in shifts. In a month she was walking around with only a slight limp without any evidence of ever being injured.

Healing often feels like disease in reverse. Instead of disease coming it, it is going out! In Reiki we have a description of the processed called "achy-Reiki." The body aches or feels pain as the adverse energy finds its way out of the body. Charging up a formerly unused meridian of energy is like a shock along a wire, and it can smart. I call it being ZAPPED. Over time increased circuitry of the body is opened. The longer you do energy work, the more ability your body will have to deliver it. Once a high capacity is developed, you will have hot hands and to be able to deliver large amounts of healing energy. You may feel a prickly sensation in your hands. The beauty of Reiki is that you always have your hands with you. On a bus, plane, or train or in an emergency, all you must do is give yourself a healing treatment. Placing your hands on each side of your neck and shoulders creates a warm healing current going down your spine. You may look like King Tut, but the energy is very healing for your spine, and it goes all the way down to heal any hemorrhoids or other localized problems as well.

As your progress into spiritual maturity many changes occur over time. Your perceptions become more acute. Hearing, sense of smell and awareness become more developed. I can only describe it as having the awareness of a hawk. Your psychic facilities appear including clairvoyance and clairaudience. You may eventually develop "eyes that see" and "ears that hear." You can suddenly hear even the planets spinning through space. Even the music of the spheres may play for your ears. Illnesses you did not even know you had become healed BEFORE they manifest. The energy from healers hands is believed to create more stem cells and therefore heal the subject from the inside out. The more you practice the longer you can keep your enlightened state. Enlightenment is simply a state of bliss where you are in balance and harmony.

How does one achieve enlightenment and a pure state of health? The answer is simple, but the path is long.

Earlier in this book we spoke of the chakra system of seven major energy portals and over 144 minor ones. If any are damaged or torn, we lose energy. (a tear over 12% can be fatal over time as immunity crashes.) If they are all open and flowing completely, we experience a greater degree of health and wellbeing. This does not mean however that they are operating to their full potential. To achieve the full potential of our chakra system all the chakras need to be joined together as one unit. They must be connected and be fully charged to full energetic capacity, like batteries connected in series. Traditionally this is called Kundalini yoga. This technique gradually raises the energy from the base of the spine and connects each chakra one by one until all are connected. This produces a chain reaction of energy like a nuclear reaction. Therefore, it must be done slowly to give the body time to adjust, adapt, and build "circuitry" of the nervous system to manage it. The Kundalini process is routinely depicted as a coiled serpent at the base of the spine.

Sometimes this energy is activated accidentally in an unprepared individual and the body circuitry becomes massively overwhelmed. It is labeled a Kundalini psychosis, where the individual develops a (hopefully) temporary insanity, until the energy is either dissipated or directed by a Kundalini yoga master.

I mention this because I experienced an unplanned Kundalini rising myself. I was reading a book one night entitled: The Return of the Serpents of Wisdom. When I read the part about the high priests of Egypt, I had the realization I was one of them. I saw myself under instruction at the great Pyramid of Giza and a lightening bolt of energy struck from the base of my spine to my heart. It was like having a heart attack and it took a few hours for me to compose myself and redirect the massive amount of energy. A Reiki master friend of mine also had a vision of us during a session. She said she saw us all dressed in white wearing gold armbands at the mystery schools along the Nile. It was a fascinating confirmation of what I had seen.

As God is unlimited healing is unlimited. We have no idea of how far it can progress. While our basic chart lists a spiritual calibration of 1,450 as the highest level of ascension the human potential is unlimited and may reach 100,000s of degrees beyond our present understanding. Some of my students have already achieved this. And once a certain level is achieved healing ability seems to double every week. Like the financial progression of $1,000 doubling 10x equals a $ million dollars, healing has the same progression.

The student however must NOT ATTEMPT TO GO TOO FAST. I speak from experience. If you push yourself too fast being an eager beaver, you will make yourself sick or land in the emergency room. If you do too much fire yoga at a time, you'll be sick for 4 days. I once met a woman at a picnic who was an Aramaic scholar and she said that to get the most power out of the healing secrets of Christ you had to say them in Aramaic. Naturally, I found such a book online and read it not thinking a thing of it. The next day I was in the emergency room with blood pressure of 225/100. I was on the couch for 3 weeks with shingles and in intense pain. So do not be an eager beaver and take heed of my mistakes. Take your time. The world will not end for a while yet. You probably have another 80 years.

Reiki has been studied scientifically and published in medical journals. If you are a health professional, you may wish to obtain a copy of Reiki in Clinical Practice and be involved in the Reiki in hospitals movement. The illustrations are extremely helpful. In the hospital setting Reiki has been confirmed to show a 30% improvement in symptoms. **Use of the Ascension Protocol and the charting procedures I have outlined can eventually lead to a 100x increase in healing power and better results can be obtained.**

For those of you who may be interested in starting your own Reiki practice I will share my personal method with you. Prior to working with a new client, I make two charts using muscle testing. The first is a **SPIRITUAL ASSESSMENT PROFILE** and the other is a **HEALING CHART**. Together they both usually run about four pages. I do this for convenience, legal issues, professionalism, and ethical standards. I always discuss with the client any issues I see and obtain their permission to do the work. Before I ever touch a person, I ask their permission to touch them and repeat this at each location on their body. Some clients may be shy at first and state that they would prefer to work on certain sensitive areas later. Clients who have never had a treatment before may be somewhat skeptical at first and they need to experience it first to be sure it is real for them. I also keep the client informed about what I am seeing or finding. I either "see" or feel issues with my hands. A buildup of 500 or more "reiki hours" of healing in any one area is indicative of a disease formation. For those healers who are not familiar with muscle testing to obtain estimates, it is extremely easy to tell if a location is affected. If an area gets hot to the hands- just keep going until it gets cool. It is that simple.

The spiritual assessment profile has the following categories:

SPIRITUAL CALIBRATION

SPIRITUAL CALIBRATION REQUIRED TO HEAL ONESELF

TARGETED HEALING NEEDED

CELLULAR HEALING NEEDED

FIRE YOGA HOURS

ENTITIES

HEART OPENNESS

DEATH POTENTIAL

STROKE POTENTIAL

CANCER POTENTIAL

CHAKRA TEARS

IMMUNE SYSTEM FUNCTIONING

INNER COSMIC ORBIT

THE SIDDHA YOGA 5 BIGGIES

BIRTH TRAUMA

PARENTAL DISAPPROVAL SYNDROME

SPECIFIC NEGATIVES

UNCONSCIOUS DEATH URGE

NEGATIVE KARMA AND ANCESTRAL KARMA

Lastly, I review with an OVERALL VIEW OF THE SUBJECT and note specific issues from the healing chart. I wrap the profile up with any past life information I may feel. Past life information may come after working with the client for a few sessions and seeing what is found once we "get in there" under the hood. The numbers obtained are merely a guide and are not set in stone. The numbers change in time both due to stress of the client and the ascension of the healer. The numbers will need to be updated prior to each session to see what progress if any has been made. Clients under extreme stress may need the same issues treated at each session to keep it under control. And they may blow out some chakras.

The assessment for fire yoga is quite important as if it is above 40 hours it may show immune system impairment. Therefore, the healer must pay particular attention to the lymph glands and immunity to revitalize each gland and area. Basic anatomy charts of the lymph glands are available on the internet and I include them with the finished typed charts, so the client knows what needs to be done. The lymph gland system is quite extensive and runs the entire body. It even draws energy from the large thigh bones in the legs. Massaging the areas while healing is amazingly effective to break up negative energy and may be twice as fast as just healing alone. Thousands of massage therapists are also Reiki masters, and this is an ideal way to treat the clients.

The HEALING CHART can pinpoint the client's issues rapidly. In Reiki we were taught to always do the head and the heart first. The heart controls the mind not the other way around. A client with high numbers on her heart is under extreme stress. Stress also tends to flow out from the heart to either side and lodge itself in the breasts, the thymus, spleen, and what I call the midpoints. Midpoints are the areas found between the collar bones and the breasts. The energy may have various levels of severity. It may feel electrical, magnetic, prickly, or very, very heavy like gout. The later is the spiritual cloud we have mentioned previously. The heavy, dark, cloudy energy is the crux of the problem and must be totally removed. Gentle massage is extremely helpful in removing it. Once the spiritual clouds and possible past life injuries are removed the cancer and disease potential of the client should be down to zero. I may add that this holistic approach to disease prevention is much more user friendly than x-rays and mammograms. Excessive radiation may cause the very condition the client is hoping to prevent. If a precancerous or cancerous condition exists then the healer must pay particular attention to the neck, armpits, thymus, spleen, etc. and once the healing of the lymphatic system is complete the client bounces back. This procedure works well with the flu or weaponized flu as well as we have discussed. The weaponized flu is still an energy imbalance and once the imbalance is corrected it is gone.

Extreme stress (or incorrect sexual practices) also tends to blow out the base chakra. Any tear above 12% can be fatal in a decade or two. The larger the tear the sooner death can occur as the immune system crashes, cancer or other diseases can get a foothold as literally one's energy "leaks out." This is extremely easy to repair like winding a clock and spinning the chakra with one's hand until it flows properly again. It used to take me about 1 minute to repair each 1% of tear. Now I can do it within one second and not even touch it. Grounding and meditation in the sand on the beach is also helpful but takes a great deal of time.

The healing ability of Reiki masters varies greatly. An experienced master may be off the chart seen earlier as the ultimate level of spiritual cali-bration. In fact, some healers and gurus are 100,000 or 200,000 more degrees above the basic Christ level. If you have read the bible, you may have read about instances where someone touched the robe of Christ and was healed. What I would label a healing "master" may have 100 times more healing capacity then a rookie Reiki master. To make an analogy this principle is like a big magnet overcoming the energy of a small magnet. Clients may heal just by being in the presence of their guru or healing master. A master or guru can remove death potential with only a hug or a kiss. It's all about energy. I like to do things as effortlessly and harmoniously as possible so I often take clients to the movies or dinner so we can sit together. I may hold their hands or place a hand on their elbow or leg. My favorite method is to do healings on the beach as this gets us both some sun, fresh salt air, and negative energy goes into the sand. Lying down together on a beach mat allows me to heal the client with my whole body and this is 10X faster than being on a table. We also watch tv at home together. Clients who need 1000s of hours of cellular healing due to car accidents and brain injuries often stay overnight and I wrap myself around them to maximize the energy. This can carry out 100 hours of equivalent reiki healing per night. The client may remain fully clothed in case you are wondering. Gandhi used to use this method all the time. Married couples can add tantric yoga healing as this is 50x more powerful than regular healing and leads to enlightenment.

Always remember that healing is unlimited as God is unlimited. If you complete healing a major life challenge just keep going. Healing is a way of life and not a one-time magic bullet. As you ascend to new levels the entire body must be healed repeatedly to adjust to the new higher level. Then you will reach greater healing ability. As you heal others the more you heal yourself as the energy flows through you.

Fire yoga takes a bit more planning, but I recommend doing it weekly until you have completed your 40 plus hours. I used to do it bi-weekly and had my computer on a portable table. Do not forget to show your appreciation to the fire for its work. Once you have completed your 40 hours try to do a quarterly tune-up and stay current. Keep disease potential from building up on your aura!!

Your friends may think you are insane for using the ascension protocol with its healing, gold powders, fire yoga, and wearing diamonds to remove negative karma. You will also stand out in a crowd if you practice mundan and shave your head for 9 months. However only by completing all the spiritual tasks will you become disease free and have an incredible immune system. There is no free lunch in the universe. The medical profession loves to sell quick fixes and mechanical means to health, but this does not do the spiritual work necessary for a better life. Nor will a vaccine remove a past life bullet hole.

THE RESERVOIR OF TRAUMA

It can be very frustrating for both the client and the healer when 15 hours of healing have been carried out and there are no noticeable results. Eventually I developed the concept of cellular healing and the reservoir of trauma. The traumatic overburden must be removed first before one can connect with the underlying cause that we are seeking to heal and remove.

As in gold mining, you have to remove tons of sand (the overburden) before you get to the gold at the bottom of the riverbed. This became clear one evening when I was working on my difficult subject when we broke through to the cause. He heated up and started to sweat. He then fell asleep on the table, and we finally began to make headway on his many injuries and surgeries.

Exactly how to proceed is best determined by the type and gravity of the situation. Time is of the essence in many conditions. The total hours are calculated to remove both the pre-existing "overburden of trauma" and the more newly formed trauma associated with the symptoms one may currently be experiencing. Completion of the healing regimen (in hours) may or not effect complete relief or remission of symptoms. The situation may require a higher spiritual calibration to unlock and remove the primary source of the condition. (Or negative karma) Old lifestyle habits that build up trauma must be replaced with more positive and nurturing habits. Healing will however remove the crushing weight of trauma being experienced and get the subject back to a neutral position where he may more easily and readily move forward physically and spiritually. Once the subject arrives at the neutral position or "square one", it is time to learn how to heal oneself and venture forth under your own power. Just three (3) hours of self-administered healing per day adds up to over a thousand hours per year. Tremendous progress can be made in a year. An annual checkup by a master healer can assist you in monitoring your progress towards your healing and spiritual goals.

To make an analogy think of an exceptionally large lake with a high dam. When the reservoir is full the water goes over the top. When the reservoir is empty several storms can occur, and the reservoir will fill back up but the dam won't be destroyed. If the reservoir is full and several huge storms come the dam might be destroyed and everything downstream will be killed. So, it is with trauma. If your lake of trauma is empty a sudden storm of trauma will only partially full your reservoir. The wise thing to do is to keep your lake of trauma empty as you'll be better able to deal with unexpected shocks and drama when they come. If you learn the ancient wisdom of Zen, your lake will never fill again. It is not the trauma itself to blame, rather it is your reaction to it. You are in control and you are the truth.

The hours of estimated healing time are not set in stone. God did not give them to me on Mt. Sinai or anything like that. Haha. They are just estimates and can change daily. There are many different healing systems and techniques. I mention Reiki most frequently as a basic system because there are one million Reiki masters in the USA. Not only are there many types of systems, but different basic types of healing energy as well. According to Dr. Eric Pearl, the developer of The Reconnection Healing Technique, there are hot Earth energies and cool astral healing frequencies and direct angelic interventions. You will have to discover for yourself which type of healing energy is best for you. The beauty of the internet is that you can experience online from Qi Gong masters like Dr & Master Sha of Toronto or from siddha masters in India at the Pillai Center. See https://drsha.com . Siddha information about healing and prosperity can be obtained at the Pillai Center in India. See: https://pillaicenter.com .

THE ORDER OF HEALING

Healing has its own divine order. I call it "the order of healing". It appears that divine intelligence knows what part of the body should be healed and in what order to insure survival. It has been my experience that the major functions of the body are healed and preserved first. The brain, heart, lungs, and kidneys are all healed first as these are most essential for the survival of the subject. The kidneys are one of the most frequently damaged organs, due to the current state of our environment. The spine, bones, and mobility issues come next. Improvement in digestion and other internal organs come later. Reproductive organs and skin conditions are not immediate survival issues and appear to heal last. Issues such as erectile dysfunction can only be reached by removing the entire pile of overburden (trauma) to get to it. Once the entire body is recharged and healed fertility improves dramatically. Smaller issues like herpes and hepatitis C disappear as the body ascends. I believe the human body is wired to shield its' fight or flight capability and hence the life and survival of the organism. Do not be surprised if your targeted healing does not go to where you wish it to go. Again, healing has its own divine intelligence, and you cannot outguess it. I was healing a clients heart once and the healing energy went straight through her body to a disc in her back. We were both incredibly surprised by this, but that is exactly what can happen.

BLOCKS TO HEALING

All illnesses have distress as their starting point, which (then) causes biological conflict. A message is sent to the brain to get to work creating an illness. As genes have inherited memories of ancient adaptations to old conflicts, illness can be considered genetic. The work of Dr. Ryke Geerd Hamer, A German physician, has been one of the first to deal with stress or trauma as a trigger to disease. Dr. Hamer used a CT scanner to identify how the brain adapts and creates illness. Traumatic evens such as the loss of a loved one, bankruptcy, or loss of quality of life alter brain waves and lead directly to alternation of the organs. Illness plays a valuable role in balancing the body of an individual to adapt to life's challenges.

Illness and disease also fulfill several spiritual, karmic, and educational functions. They ALWAYS occur for a reason and not at the random whim of God or nature. **THE MIND CREATED THE ILLNESS OR DISEASE FOR A SPECIFIC PURPOSE.** Knowing that "inner work" is needed to resolve illness is one of the biggest keys to its' removal or neutralization. One must become attuned to the cycles of the Earth, life, and death, as all things are temporary. The word therapeutic derives from the ancient "Therapeutae of Egypt, (and the Essenes) which means "physicians of the soul." Complete healing requires total healing of the body, mind, and spirit. The reason some illnesses are unresolved is that the healing just stops too soon.

It is necessary to put into plain terms why disease is with us: **people become overly attached to their diseases and even define themselves as one who has a particular disease.** For example, members of Alcoholics

Anonymous introduce themselves as, "Hello, I'm Robert, I'm an alcoholic". While being in the truth can be helpful at times, seeing yourself as a co-creator with God is more useful. The same scenario is true with diabetics, drug users, or persons with cancer. They all define themselves as persons with this or that disease. I would like to remind you that you are NOT your disease: you are a just a human being. As the mind created it the mind can uncreate it.

There is nothing better than a crippling disease to either spiritually educate, karmically balance or simply punish your wayward mother. If you need to keep your husband from divorcing you and walking out just roll the car over three times and maybe catch yourself on fire for some extra drama. That will slow him down for three years nursing you back to health. Who would pass up the opportunity for a multi-million-dollar lawsuit and the opportunity to blame someone else for your life just to be well? If humans run low on their stockpile of diseases, they are forced to invent something else to use as a vehicle to accomplish their desires. Polio used to cripple million s of people per year until it was virtually eradicated. Therefore, the human psyche called in extra cases of MS and car accidents to fulfill the need to be crippled. If you want to dissolve a disease, you must first determine its purpose.

Is it an "oh poor me" disease, or an "get out of work that I hate disease", or just the usual "I need more love and attention sort of disease? How about "my shit life disease"? Sometimes however the disease, illness or accident is THE ANGELS HOOK. In this scenario you signed up for this before you were born because you knew you would never make the spiritual progress necessary in this life unless you had an INCENTIVE to do so. Life threatening scenarios require a decision to move forward or die. Been there!! All diseases have a reason. The spiritual reasons for most common diseases are cataloged in Christian Fleche's book entitled The Bio-genealogy Sourcebook: Healing the Body by Resolving Traumas of the Past. If you don't heal the cause, you have accomplished nothing. Even if you had a magic bullet that instantly cured a disease, if the individual wasn't done with it yet and totally released it then he can instantly make another one to replace it. Or maybe just get hit by a bus. When I worked with a client called Abby, I sorted out her past life experiences of murder, torture and hatred. Then I whispered in her ear, "JUST LET IT GO!" The next time she saw me at the hospital she said, "It feels like a tremendous weight has been lifted from me." Two weeks later she was released from the hospital and went home to her family. She had been in intensive care for over 6 months.

Eradicating a disease is a much bigger chore than most people imagine. To get finally, completely, totally rid of one you must treat body, mind, and spirit. Medicine and healing got divorced sometime during the period known as the enlightenment. Rational men of science wanted nothing to do with the spiritual hocus-pocus and religious mumbo-jumbo. They wanted only hard science and facts. The time has come for medicine and healing to kiss and make up.

CHAPTER 5

WATER WATER EVERYWHERE. THE HUNZAS SECRET.

IT IS AN OLD SAYING that there is water water everywhere, not a drop fit to drink. Unfortunately, in the modern "civilized" world that is quite true. Our water is not fit to drink. Tap water is merely slow suicide. The physics of water is the key to health and longevity. It is the key to the cause of fatalities from the flu and weaponized flu aka Covid-19. The bonding angles of oxygen can be destroyed by extreme stress, toxins, emf, and poor diet. When the bonding angles are destroyed the perfect crystalline structure of the cells collapse, toxins can no longer be removed, oxygen can no longer attach itself to hemoglobin in the blood and the subject is asphyxiated. Medical intervention in the form of aggressive ventilation can then cause pneumonia and the demise of the patient. Therefore, if we look at the root cause of asphyxia many lives can be saved.

You may not be interested in fathering children at over the age of 100 or living past a minimum of 130 years, but if you do then you need a copy of Dr. Patrick Flannigan's Elixir of the Ageless. The text is a bit technical, but well worth reading. It is a major scientific breakthrough that few people are aware of.

For over a decade America's most distinguished scientists, Doctor Patrick Flanigan tried to discover the secrets of the Hunza people in Pakistan. The Hunzas all seemed to live beyond 100 years of age, with some as old as 150. Patrick Flanigan eventually discovered that the milky white glacial water from the mountains was their secret. The water was full of small micro-particles of minerals, and this allowed a greater accumulation of electricity to gather around them. Later he was able to reproduce these micro clusters of energy or colloids in the lab. Eventually he created Crystal Energy or Flanigan colloids. Doctor Flanigan found that the higher the electrical potential or Zeta potential as he called it, the more beneficial the water was to health. Colloids form long electrically charged chains, holding as much as 40,000 volts. They form in series like little batteries and the electrical charge helps the water remove toxins from the body. The result of this high electrical charge in the water is a 500% improvement in vitamin absorption and a greatly increased lifespan. Crystal Energy also pulls your body pH in the right direction. More alkaline if you need it, more acid if you need it. And daily use of crystal energy acts as a natural chelator pulling out heavy metals and other toxins.

Flanagan has continued his research on the healing waters of the world for over three decades. His work has focused primarily on what mechanisms participate in hydrating the cells of the body. He found that negatively charged hydrogen ions are responsible for delivering water to the cells. It is the combination of oxygen and hydrogen in an electrically charged structure that is needed for the body's energy and fuel. **Hydrogen restructures blood**, separating the cells so that they can efficiently remove toxins and free radicals that destroy cellular DNA. As free radicals and oxidants are a cause of cellular deterioration and aging the effects of rehydrating the cells is dramatic. Hydrogen is the key to life, death, and aging.

Normally we get our hydrogen for water, fruits, and vegetables. Due to all the hazards of civilized life, chemical agriculture, food processing, stress, etc. we do not get enough hydrogen in our diets to maintain a healthy balance of our cellular structure. Our cells become oxidized and full of free radicals. We wear out ourselves like an old rusty pipe. The addition of silica hydride from MegaHydrate reverses the process and rehydrates our cells and rebuilds their energy carrying capacity called Zeta Potential. One dose of MegaHydrate has more antioxidant power than hundreds of glasses of fresh vegetable and fruit juices, broccoli, Brussels sprouts, leafy greens, and other fruits foods rich in antioxidants to prevent free radical damage. In short MegaHydrate can be considered an anti-aging pill. It also supplies **natural pain relief** from headaches, sore muscles, and inflammation of the joints. Normally it takes about a month to rehydrate the cells using MegaHydrate. Crystal Energy and MegaHydrate are available online. I take Crystal Energy daily.

CHAPTER 6

PERFECT SCIENCE WATER

A MIRACLE HAPPENED IN THE late 1980s, but only a few people ever heard about it outside of the FBI, CIA and other high government agencies. Officials in Russia and eight other countries at once began to investigate this new discovery. The Turkish government built a new $48 million dollar plant to produce 100,000 gallons a day of what is called Perfect Science Water." This super ionized water with 3 extra electrons on its outer orbit is like no other water on Earth. Due to its molecular structure, it is alive and has "God-Consciousness". It has the uncanny ability to turn toxic substances into proteins and amino acids. It works on chemical dumps, polluted rivers and bays, and even nuclear waste. It can cleanup a polluted river or lake in as little as 3-4 days. Just a couple of gallons of Perfect Science water cleaned up Izmit Bay near Istanbul. It went clear. Tests were done on a swimming pool of sewage. In less than a few hours it was clear. (www.perfectscience.com) . You may also order Perfect Science Waters for your own detoxification.

Perfect Science Water can be used to clean up toxic sites, mining wastes and polluted agricultural land. It even puts out forest fires and chemical fires in a very rapid fashion.

Perfect Science Water may be the best toxin cleaner ever developed. We will see as times goes on. Its potential for use in the human body is immense. There is already anecdotal evidence of its usefulness in fighting degenerative diseases such as cancer, heart disease, AIDS, and diabetes. An aids clinic is planned for Haiti to evaluate its effectiveness. (2008) Much more testing and clinical studies are needed.

Scientist at the University of Georgia discovered the "every cell in our body that is diseased, or that is harmed in one way, or another is surrounded by UNSTRUCTURED WATER." Unstructured water is missing electrons in the outer orbit. Therefore, supplying these missing electrons returns the cells to a "structured" state and hence eliminates the foundation of disease!!

Also, the use of clustered water "appears to be a definite step forward in allowing consciousness inside the human body to emerge faster!!"

Under the microscope clustered water looks like tiny snowflakes with structured hexagonal patterns. You can think of clustered water as "liquid electrons." And the more you have, the better. Every function in the body is either pushed or pulled by electromagnetic action, like tiny magnets moving stuff on a conveyor belt. Without this electrical activity cellular functions slow down and the body gets sludged up. And that is the primary cause of all our problems.

Only clean running water has the minerals, energy, and "life" in it to keep your body healthy. Tap water is DEAD. It can be full of sewage, toilet paper and chlorine. If it is pure, then all the minerals and electrical energy are also removed. (The reverse osmosis method. Dr. Patrick Flanigan calls drinking tap water a slow form of suicide. Today's tap water is yesterday's toilet. Dr. Flanigan has discovered everything in tap water from cesium 6, made famous in the film Erin Brockovich, to rocket fuel. Your body is made mostly of water and if you need to regain your health you need to first rebuild your cellular system with structured super-ionized water. Prana or energy and water combined are the structure of our DNA.

CHAPTER 7

THE NEW GARDENERS

IT IS OFTEN JOKINGLY SAID that "we treat our soil like dirt!!" The soil is however a living, breathing, spiritual entity full of living organisms, enzymes, and minerals all bonded together in a dynamic biosphere. This all takes place in, and is influenced by, a local and cosmic electromagnetic environment.

Agribusiness has turned this sacred ground into killing fields solely for the sake of profit. There are over 2,300 cancer causing chemicals sprayed upon our food, some of which are so lethal that one drop absorbed through the skin causes death. The chemicals designed to kill insects kill the soil as well. Farmers are going bankrupt in record numbers because their reliance upon expensive poisonous sprays and synthetic fertilizers simply does not work in the long run.

There are other ways. Organic gardening has been popularized in this country by Robert Rodale. Biodynamic gardening (www.biodynamics.com) was originated by Rudolf Steiner in Austria in 1924, has developed a highly effective approach to gardening. Spiritual gardeners such as Peter Caddy from Findhorn, Scotland (www.findhorn.org) and Michelle Small Wright of Perelandra Farms in Jeffersonville, Va. (www.perelandra-ltd.com) have reintroduced gardening in its original spiritual form. These later approaches consider the sacredness of all life and work with respect for and cooperation with the elemental forces of nature.

Foods grown in the sacred manner are vibrantly alive: full of energy. They are highly structurally organized on a cellular electromagnetic level. When eaten raw, the largest amount of food energy is released into the body through a process called "subtle organizing energy fields" (SOEFs) These energy fields are "coded" like a computer disk and help direct the food energy to its proper location and purpose through a process of electromagnetic attraction. Unenlightened growing practices result in weak, inferior, and often toxic food. (and ultimately a weak, inferior, toxic population). Cooking practices further destroy its vitality as heat destroys the electromagnetic bonds of the SOEFs. Doctors at the 'Shanghai College of Traditional Chinese Medicine have discovered that foods cooked in glass or ceramics were most effective in inhibiting cancer growth. As they say in computer programming, "garbage in-garbage out". Incorrect thinking, growing, and eating habits result in a loss of energy throughout the body. This in turn creates a "brown out effect" where vital bodily functions are taken "off the circuit" in an attempt to save the most vital functions and life. Imbalance of energy within the body are the unguard gates through which disease invades the body. Correct dietary, mental, and healing practices can "super charge" the body and makes it extremely resistant, if not totally immune to all diseases.

Organic gardening techniques supply the proper nutritional "structure" in an electromagnetic environment that allow nutrients to be fully utilized by the body. Compost is a natural chelating agent that promotes absorption of essential elements, trace elements, and minerals. Using "rock dust", such as Azomite (www.azomite.com) can add 70 different minerals and trace elements for absorption. A technique called "sonic bloom" enhances mineral and trace element absorption by as much as 700%. Protein content can be improved, even doubled. As Christopher Bird has so eloquently pointed out in his **SECRETS OF THE SOIL.**, **THERE WERE VIRTUALLY**

NO DEGENERATIVE DISEASES IN THIS COUNTRY UNTIL THE ADVENT OF CHEMICAL AGRICULTURE AT THE TURN OF THE CENTURY! Degenerative disease accounted for only 1% of all deaths in 1902 but accounted for 60% by 1948. As early as 1936 US Senate hearings were being conducted as per the poor state of America's soils. Except for a few enlightened organic gardeners, the downward trend continues with disastrous results to the public health.

According to a Seattle Times article (www.rense.com/health/toxicchem.htm" radioactive and toxic chemicals are frequently sold as farm fertilizer. In the USA, there are no regulations set on toxic and radioactive waste in farm fertilizers. Steel mills, pulp mills, smelters, and even medical and municipal waste companies find "recycling" their waste as fertilizer saves them money. "Use of industrial waste as a fertilizer ingredient is a growing national phenomenon, The Times reported." Can there be any doubt why humans and animals aren't as healthy as they were 100 years ago? You can safely and easily find out whether you have been affected by this trend by sending a sample of your hair for analysis. The cost is approximately $170.00. And throw your toothpaste away while you are at it. Its full of toxic waste also!

Dr. Joel Wallach, N.D. has contributed significantly to our knowledge of mineral deficiency as a major cause of death. He is the author of the best-selling **DEAD DOCTORS DON'T LIE** and **RARE EARTHS-FORBIDDEN CURES**. He was nominated for a Nobel Prize in 1991 for his stunning discoveries in the use of trace minerals to prevent catastrophic diseases in the newborn. You can obtain his books on minerals, aurio tapes, and vitamin and miner line at: (www.wallachonline.com". Consumption of the 90 different minerals you need brings very noticeable improvement to your overall health.

Perhaps the most critically missing ingredient in commercial chemically produced food is nitrogen. Chemical techniques do not make nitrogen available in a usable form for use in the body. Organic techniques such as crop rotation and lightening both affix nitrogen to the soil where it can be absorbed by the food grown in it. According to Gaston Naessens, cancerous cells crave nitrogen and when it is supplied in sufficient quantities they dissolve! This may explain why Chinese, Egyptian, Mayan, and Inca agriculturists went to such great pains to add more electromagnetic energy to their soils, to improve soil fertility, and to promote human and animal vitality and longevity.

The most basic problem with chemical agriculture is that it is incompatible with the true nature of the Earth. It ignores all the true rules of physics and of the universe to make a quick buck. Like many other systems purveyed by hucksters and bankers, chemical agriculture is a scam. A Ponzi scheme to trick the Earth and farmers into producing more for less money. It produces less for more money and creates a tidal wave of death and disease in its wake. It would cost an average family of 4 over $1,000 a month in vitamin and mineral supplements just to replenish half of what is missing in our foods. The problem is the consumers do not know what they're missing. And many will never realize it until they have a life-threatening disease. What they are missing is best classified as super conductors of energy. These superconductors are known as monatomic metallic elements. Regardless of how many vitamins and minerals you have, you cannot live without M-state elements in your diet. M-state products have not made it into use in agriculture yet except on an experimental basis. You can judge the results yourself of Barry Carter's experiments with walnut trees. Zero Point Technologies has stated that, "There is a super health and wellness revolution on the horizon" and I totally agree. (www.zptech.com)

RECREATING THE GARDEN OF EDEN

The biblical garden of Eden is believed to have been the delta area where the rivers Tigris and Euphrates meet in modern Iraq. We must ask ourselves what is so special about river deltas that would make agriculture in such an area a veritable paradise on earth? In other words what creates a perfect soil for agriculture? Previously we discussed how the white milky glacial melt water in the Hunzas lands brought down a wealth of colloidal minerals in a highly charged electrical matrix. Obviously, the richer the minerals in the area, the better the resulting soil will be. High volcanic mountain ranges, rich in gold, silver, copper, or other minerals ALSO have their M-state isotopes of these same elements. Delta areas made of high concentrations of M-state minerals are the richest soils in the world, both for agriculture and for healing. One such area is located 40 miles south of Lima, Peru. M-state minerals from the Andes bless the area with a healing mud that is extremely popular with the local inhabitants. As minerals are absorbed through the skin, the inhabitants cover themselves in mud daily for about 30 days. This method is extremely popular as a low-cost method of treating skin conditions. As each stream in the area has different minerals, some streams work better on certain diseases and ailments than others. Any river system carrying M-state and glacial melt from high volcanic mountains is a candidate for healthful agriculture and healing. Volcanic hot springs in the Andes, such as the ones in Calca, (near Cuzco) may be the source of these minerals and are highly beneficial. Many islands in the world are volcanic in origin and are a wonderful place to look for hot springs. The Hawaiian chain is the best place in the USA to look for mineral-bearing hot springs. The volcanic island nation of Iceland holds the record for having the longest-lived people. Yoga master Sondra Ray leads spiritual tours to Iceland and India. (http://sondraray.com)

We can naturally recreate these Edenic conditions using M-state bearing sands, M-state sprays, bio-dynamic gardening, rock dust (Azomite), and placement of large crystalline stones of certain vibrations. We have seen how walnuts the size of tennis balls can be achieved with M-state sprays (C-11 from Ocean Alchemy). This seems to hold true for other plant species as well. An M-state grown pepper plant grew 10 times the size of its control. The time has come to plant entire farms using M-state sprays and soils. I believe the results will be dramatically superior to anything chemical agriculture ever produced. Personally, I believe M-state minerals are the missing link in human health. M-state minerals are what can help humanity reach its true God-given potential. Dr. Patrick Flannigan has already proven that the simple addition of colloids can increase vitamin absorption by 500%. Imagine what would happen if everything we ate was full of the proper amount of

M-state and colloids!! One farmer reported growing ears of corn 22 inches long using water from a living water machine. The use of living water and ormus products opens a whole new dimension in agriculture.

For starters, I believe the obesity rate would decline dramatically. I believe that part of the overeating scenario is the body's quest for sufficient energy and hydration. These are terribly lacking in today's foods. In 1965, Dr. Nilo Cairo and A. Brinckmann came to the same conclusion as I did that colloidal gold was the one remedy against obesity.

Foods rich in M-state, deserve a larger role in the common diet. Grape plants have roots that can extend down 40 feet and gather more M-state minerals than nearly any other plant. This explains the "French Paradox", as to why the French have long life spans despite their extraordinarily rich, fatty diets. **Concord grapes have enough of the antioxidant resveratrol to inhibit the reproduction of the flu virus by 90%. If we could get a better picture of the M-state ingredients of grapes, it may be possible to create an effective countermeasure for the flu virus.** I believe that a doubling of human lifespan is possible solely through a complete understanding of the health benefits of M-state minerals. The Hunzas can do it, why can't we? (note you can buy resveratrol for about $20.00 to supplement your diet.)

The bottom line on natural foods and herbs is that there is indeed an herbal or whole food remedy for nearly every disease or condition under the sun. Many have been used for thousands of years with no ill effects. I have supplied a number of additional books in the bibliography section to assist the reader in this regard. You have all seen the impressive Madison Avenue ad campaigns for drugs on TV. Some guy comes on offering wonderful news that you can reduce your cholesterol level by over 30% just by taking their magic drug for $100 in cash. What they do not tell you is that you could do the same thing by eating an onion! Yeah, an onion! Or garlic. A daily diet of walnuts will cut your cholesterol by 100%. My VA doctor was shocked!! The same story goes for just about every other miracle drug out there. There is a natural alternative that works as well without the side effects. Stressed out? Do not take a dangerous mind-altering drug: eat an apple and detoxify. See your naturopathic physician. He can help you sort it all out. Get a tan!! And finally, I believe that once more knowledge is gained about the daily requirements of Ormus metallic elements there will indeed be a revolution in growing practices and dietary consumption. A new dawn of "super food" is about to rise and our medicine cabinet will look a whole lot different when they do. I am talking about foods and medicines WITHOUT toxins that help, not kill, the patient. Have not convinced you yet? Then men consider this: toxins and plastics can mimic estrogen and make your penis small. And you can get what my thirteen-year-old daughter calls, "man boobs". Plus, you get fat of course. Ha ha Are you convinced yet? I hope so. **GET TO KNOW YOUR FARMER NOT YOUR DOCTOR.**

THE PHILOSOPHERS STONE

Monatomic or Ormus (High Orbital spin rate) metallic elements may be nature's most bizarre, unusual, and ultimately most useful elements on the face of the Earth. While you may never have heard of ormus (also spelled Ormes) materials or as it was called "The Philosophers Stone" by the ancients, without them you would probably cease to exist. It has also been known as "manna from heaven", and "the universal cure", and "the holy grail" to name a few. While gold is a perfect conductor of electricity, Ormus gold is a "super-conductor" of the highest magnitude. The super conducting ability of monatomic elements has any number of radical and fascinating applications.

The high orbital invisible "stealth elements" of gold and platinum group metals can do amazing things including a disappearing into other dimensions. Just a partial list of discoveries will give an indication of future developments in metals refining and agriculture.

First, our very brain tissue itself is by dry weight, composed of 5% monatomic iridium and rhodium. The implications for creating a few geniuses or treating brain dysfunctions are immense. **Ormus iridium affects the pituitary gland in a way that reactivates the body's junk DNA and underused parts of the brain. Feeling stupid today?** Take a little iridium and rhodium and call me in the morning. Colloidal gold has been proven to raise I.Q. as much as 20 points in 30 days. Certainly the thing to have for finals week. White powdered gold (M-state) can be used to connect the **GOLDEN TRIANGLE** of the upper chakras and open **THE CRYSTAL CAVE** of latent brain power and alleged junk DNA with incredible results.

Bristol Meyers Squibb found that when single ruthenium atoms are placed at each end of a short strand of DNA it becomes **10,000 times more conductive! It becomes in effect a superconductor. The use of platinum, iridium and ruthenium atoms in the treatment of cancer, corrects the deformed cancer cells. Monatomic gold and platinum group metals dismantle incorrect DNA and rebuild the DNA again correctly. They activate the endocrine system and pineal gland in a way that heightens awareness and aptitude to extraordinary levels.**

Increased melatonin from the pineal gland affects the immune system and heightens energy, stamina, physical tolerance levels and sleep patterns. All of these bodily enhancements lead to heightened self-awareness, inner vision, psychic phenomena, and intuitive vision.

Ormus products have been used successfully to treat leukemia, AIDS, and cancer. They have been used on MS, Lou Gehrig's Disease, MD, and even arthritis. They even get rid of KS (Kaposi Sarcoma). Ormus materials are so potent that a mere 2 mg injection raises white cell count from 2,500 to 6,500 in 2 hours. Stage 4 cancer patients who have taken Ormus materials orally were totally cancer free in 45 days. The mass production of Ormus products would seem to have the potential to eliminate the current corrupt cancer industry. Which may explain why you have not heard of them?

Although understanding why Ormus does what it does is a matter for conjecture among nuclear particle physicists and alchemists, the lower-level formulae are not hard or expensive to make. In fact, the wet methods can produce Ormus from rather ordinary sea water, or well water for under $45.00.

Alchemy means "higher science" and is the forerunner of the word chemistry. Alchemy is the missing key to the mystical experiences of Western religions and Western science. The "stone that the builders rejected" is the foundation of Egyptian, Greek, Gnostic, Christian, Hebrew, and Islamic religions. In the East, manna or the Philosophers Stone is the means for creating the SOMA: The ELIXIR OF IMMORTALITY. The Soma are actually hormonal secretions from the roof of one's mouth created by the activations of the various latent glandular functions.

The Egyptian Pharaohs were the first to use white gold powders for health and longevity. Then came the Greek philosophers in Alexandria, Egypt, with its great library, was the hotbed of alchemy and learning. Adepts from all over the world traveled to Alexandria to learn its secrets.

One such group that knew the secrets of practical alchemy was the Essenes. Their monastery was located on the Dead Sea, which is a tremendous source of minerals and Ormus materials. The Dead Sea salts produce one of the highest concentrations of M-state gold. The precipitate contains approximately 70% gold and can be ordered from Ocean Manna. The most well-known Essene was of course Jesus the Nazarene. Jesus was a "Master of the Craft," not a master craftsman or carpenter. This I believe was a deliberate misconception, not a clerical error. A "Master of the Craft" is one who has mastered the art and science of alchemy and metallurgy. Jesus used and possibly made the ancient Egyptian white gold powder formulas as used by the pharaohs. Jesus was a guardian of the ancient knowledge and therefore the scientific knowledge Jesus had was immense. Mary Magdalene, the high priestess, and wife of Jesus was also an accomplished alchemist and apparently one of the first women to write a book on alchemy. She was known in France simply as Mary the Jewess. She was also an inventor, creating such things as the hot ash box, the dung box, and the double boiler still in use today. After a long life of prayer and meditation in the caves of the south of Marseille, France she was interred in the Chapel at Ile de Mary, France. (Gardener cites St. Maximus Monastery.)

Knowledge is the antidote to enslavement and therefore the threat to all authoritarian governments. What we commonly think of the names for the people in the bible are spiritual titles. "A Mary", "A Joseph", and "A Christ" (meaning both savior and fire as in master of tantric energy.) are all titles given to individuals who have gained proficiency and knowledge of a certain degree. These titles were also used to keep the true identities secret and therefore safe from persecution. What therefore is most relevant is how do we begin these studies? Without knowing where to begin it would be difficult or impossible to attain "the Christ within" or THE SECOND COMING OF CHRIST. It is this Second Birth" that is enormously important. That is why so much effort has been exerted to keep this knowledge secret. Anyone can aspire to become "A Christ", "A master of the craft" or a tantric master.

Enough ancient knowledge and practices have survived in the East and in the West. The problem is, despite improved communications media, the left hand rarely knows of what the right hand is doing. As much of the ancient knowledge stays secret, there is a HUGE information gap between East and West.

The potential to eradicate disease totally is immense. Likewise, the potential to create a new world economy, without booms and busts is also clear. What currently prevents this is that "knowledge" is too compartmentalized and specialized and not in the public domain and awareness. Historically, whenever any new form of technological or philosophical outbreak is turned loose, society is transformed. The industrial revolution at once comes to mind. As it changed the entire world as indeed every new major invention or concept does. That is why the "powers that be", try to keep all the knowledge under wraps, so it does not break free from their control. No power can keep knowledge secret indefinitely. It will always look to escape despite all the book burning and authoritarian governments of this world. **If this knowledge can reach the public domain, then a new golden age will begin.**

CHAPTER 8

ENERGY: THE GOOD, THE BAD, AND THE UGLY

EVERY ENERGY SOURCE IS A potential pathway to health and eventually enlightenment if used correctly.

Up until now we've mostly talked about beneficial forces of energy for healthful living and spiritual unfoldment. Indian Vedic architecture and Chinese Feng Shue deal with increasing the positive harmonious aspect of a home or workplace and diminishing the unhealthy, inharmonious forces of nature.

In 1879 Thomas Edison invented the light bulb and shortly thereafter the first hydroelectric plants were built to electrify homes. This was hailed as a great achievement at the time. Behind the scenes however was a raging battle over the health and safety issues of electricity. Edison supported that only D/C was safe, and that A/C was extremely dangerous for the human body to be exposed to. The big money interests were behind Tesla's and Westinghouse's inventions, A/C and the benefits of large industrial capacity electricity. In short there was money to be made! THEY lampooned Edison in the press as an old fool, although we know now that Edison was totally correct. A/C is dangerous! The cycles of A/C too closely mimic the heart. The magnetic currents created can disrupt the activity of the aura and if left untreated can create an environment for degenerative diseases such as cancer and diabetes. As medical science does not often recognize energy "pollution" for what it is, the patient is sent home to die with a pain pill.

Helmut Ziehe became interested in the effects of electricity when he developed diabetes and a host of other health problems. He eventually discovered that the magnetic forces created by A/C are especially harmful during sleep, when the body defenses are down. So, he put a switch on his fuse box and began to turn off the current to his bedroom during the night. He replaced his electric clock with a battery powered one. Within a few months, his diabetes and other health complications vanished. The culprit was apparently the electric clock near his head.

Helmut Ziehe because so fascinated with what he had discovered he founded the Bau-Biology Institute and developed a course of study to certify home "inspectors" who could ferret out the harmful situations in a home.

Fast forward 152 years and now we have a vast proliferation of electrical devices no one can live without. Everything in our homes is electric. Washer, dryer, stove, refrigerator, microwave, TV, kindles, smart meters, smart homes, alarm clocks, computer, printers, wi-fi router, hair dryers, and even the toothbrush. Might even have a security system. The list is endless. All emitting emfs. And let's not forget the cell phones which are biologically attached to our children!!

So, lets begin with we are all living in an electrical smog and few homes have devices or protection to neutralize it. An overload of electro-magnetic fields can damage your aura or your electrical body and create diseases such as cancer and diabetes. Long term continuous use of a cell phone for 15 minutes a day for 10 years leads to brain tumors. Damage to your DNA and calcium cycle does occur. When your cell phone is out of range it increases its signal 10,000 times to find a tower. The science behind emf pollution can get rather complicated. Dr. Joseph Marcola has written a New York Times best seller called EMF*D, 5G, Wi-Fi and cell Phones: Hidden Harms and How to Protect Yourself. Over use of a cell phone is the equivalent of 1,500 X-Rays. Therefore you need to protect yourself with EMF blocking equipment and clothing to block 99.% of radiation. You can start small with a Faraday bag for your cell phone at $20. And one for your Wi-Fi router. You can add clothing and blankets infused with silver monthly until full protection is obtained. An EMF Harmony wristband is $80.00.

5G cell tower radiation (and satellite radiation) however is at the heart of the Covid hoax, and the goal is to have small substations or repeaters every 100 meters. Millions of towers and satellites are to be built to blanket the entire Earth. This may literally kill the planet and everything on it. Part of the reason the bad guys wanted lockdowns was so they could install equipment on every public building, school, and church away from prying eyes. Therefore, if you want to enjoy the benefits of 5G have a fiber optic connection to your home instead and ensure your community does the same. Otherwise, you may be exposed to fatal concentrations of EMFs. Urban environments may have already passed the point of no return and EMFs can enter through your widows. Hurricane shutters painted with EMF blocking paint should solve this problem. And you can paint the interior of your home as well. You can obtain EMF blocking paint from www.emrss.com (310) 746-3686 or get the latest list from www.toolsfor freedom.com.

Cell phone towers have a line-of-sight range or the curvature of the Earth. Therefore, their range is limited to about 7 miles unless they're on a mountaintop. A rural setting out of range is the best solution and it is more defensible. EMFs from satellites can be a problem, but thick walls and trees absorb most of it. To be sure just test your home and if the reading is too high just use EMF paint and plenty of EMF materials.

Billionaire developer and former President Donald Trump has embraced the principles of Feng Shui in his buildings, but he is the exception.

Many thousands of offices are now classified as "sick buildings" and have a syndrome named after them. However, for most people, the home is the most dangerous place you can be. If you are ill, check out The Natural House Book., Bau-Biology, or Feng Shui. Natural log cabins are a perfect alternative because they "breathe" and don't build up harmful electrical charges. Hospitals may be the most dangerous places on the planet. A hot spring, spa type environment with log cabin cottages would supply a more nearly ideal environment for patients to recuperate. Or cottages on the ocean in a sunny locale. Go to the beach or forest and ground yourself as often as possible and learn a form of energy healing such as Reiki to **keep your aura healthy**. Remember that Covid is an energy imbalance and not an infectious agent.

EPILOGUE

HISTORY IS A GREAT TEACHER, but only for those who pay attention to its lessons. Few predicted the aggression of Adolph Hitler when he invaded Poland on September 1st, 1939. World leaders still had their heads in the sand as he invaded France on May 10th, 1940. Resistance fighters even infiltrated Auschwitz by being arrested so they could report on conditions there. But no one listened. In my former life I was one of the first to liberate a Nazi concentration camp. It was an unspeakable horror.

History repeats itself and we are currently in the same position as Europe in the 1930s. As guns and bullets are expensive a new means of biological warfare and mass deception have been deployed. Covid-19 is the Trojan Horse being used to bring in the 4th Reich. The war on terrorism got old, so now it's the war on germs. This a war of information. The New World Order calls it the Green New Deal, but it is the same deal as usual for world domination. The same old chestnut only the players have changed. If you did not like the 3rd Reich, you sure as hell will not like the 4th Reich. Hitler escaped to Argentina during the battle for Berlin. If you miss the bad old days under the Fuhrer, his ranch in Patagonia is currently for sale. I would estimate that Hitler lived to about 86 years of age and therefore had a couple of decades to plan the coming 4th Reich in his extremely comfortable retirement.

Canadian scientists tell their government that the Coronavirus is "The Greatest hoax ever perpetuated on an unsuspecting public." It appears a glass of concord grape juice is more effective than any vaccine, but the Boys from Brazil are always pushing vaccines to keep us safe. If you buy into this nonsense and open the door to relocation of "HIGH RISK" people, then the door will never be closed again until there are no more people to transport. Tennessee governor Bill Lee has signed executive order #83 (section 18) allowing the state National Guard to transport those alleged to have covid to treatment camps called isolation facilities run by FEMA. As you may recall if you've read part 1, in a national emergency FEMA camps will be run by Blood Alley (Manhattan) United Nations troops, i.e. the Chinese. This is the second state to authorize their National Guard to transport alleged covid patients. The problem is the common cold is a Coronavirus and current testing methods can literally be spun to target anyone. If you live in a blue Democratic state, you're already 2.5 times more likely to die. I suggest boycotting any governor in support of transportation or relocation of its citizens. The United Nations website advertised for DISARMAMENT, DEMOBILIZATION AND REINTEGRATION OFFICERS last year, so I guess they have everyone ready.

Those who are unvaccinated may be the first targets and labeled high risk as the pandemic scam is totally political. Those with PhDs have the lowest vaccination rate. Currently black Americans are only 23% vaccinated. So, they may be the first to go to the camps followed by Republicans at 50% unvaccinated. Democrats are rated at 98% vaccine compliance so they will be the first to die from the vaccines in 1-3 years. By September 15, 2021, all 2 million members of the military are to be vaccinated. And many companies such as American Airlines want 100% vaccination as a term of employment. The whole point of this rush to vaccination is to destroy American infrastructure to make it easier for conquest. If the planes don't fly, the trains don't run, the food isn't grown, the food isn't transported, we run out of gas, run out of water, the lights go off then the whole system collapses. Then all the banks close as well. In the event the targeted fatality projections aren't reached, all the bad guys must do is spray nanoparticles and more poisons with their 1,000 plus chemtrail fleet to get the numbers back on track. I think this is already happening in Florida as Governor DeSantis is opposed to lockdowns and health passports. There has been a wave of new covid cases and high fatalities. Funeral homes must rent refrigerated trailers to contain the excess of bodies. I know this as I helped transport them. We have time to avert this danger if we nip it in the bud. **Just remember that if you are on the front lines like me, if you complete the Ascension Protocol and develop Universal Immunity you not only save yourself and your loved ones, but you save America also.**

However, the powers that be do not understand the American character like I do. Garry Wills summed it up beautifully in <u>John Wayne's America</u>. "Our basic myth is that of the frontier. Our hero is the frontiersman. To become urban is to break the spirit of man. Freedom is out on the plains under endless sky. **A pent-in American ceases to be an American**." (5) page 320. In short American's aren't cut out for captivity and will resist.

Fortunately, there is still some time to wake up the people to the dangers of the new improved worldwide holocaust that lies ahead. 100 years ago, there was no warning. Now there is. Do not be fooled by the devil's silvery tongue. Unless you take your blinders off, you will find yourself in the same position as the French Resistance in WWII. Fortunately, we have resistance fighters already coming forward. Dr. Simone Gold and America's Frontline Doctors, Dr. Vladimir Zelenko (Zelenko Protocol), Dr. Joseph Mercola, Dr. Vernon Coleman, Dr. Richard Fleming, Dr. Judy Mikovits, Dr. Sherri Tenpenny, Gregory Lessing Garrett, Alex Berenson, and the ever-awesome Mike Adams: the Health Ranger @ <u>www.brighteon.com</u> . I am sure I will be added to the list of "notorious antivaxxers" and the "disinformation dozen" in a few days after publication. Who knew being healthy would become a subversive activity? We are told Covid-19 is contagious and the only hope is for vaccines and world government to save us 2.3 million times a month by the controlled fake news media. Don't believe it. As the methods of control are far more devious the deck is stacked against us, but light always wins over darkness.

All the rats are fleeing the ship. Have you noticed all the major CEOS have resigned and are selling their homes? They are all moving to the

Caribbean and building fortified residences. This is an indicator of riots in the streets and potentially civil war. Edgar Cayce predicted a period of unrest that would last several months and recommended residing in Canada on the farm until it is over. He also predicted a time when the economy would be so bad that half the women in America would be forced into prostitution to feed their children. 40% of Americans may already be on food stamps. The trends are noticeably clear. 100 million Americans may die from the vaccine alone.

The vision of our Founding Fathers has been trampled into the dust. Our Constitution and Bill of Rights have been under attack since day one. The ink was barely dry on the Bill of Rights before Alexander Hamilton helped establish a Rothschild bank- the First Bank of the United States. When President Andrew Jackson vetoed their charter there was a failed plot to assassinate him. The trail of corruption and profiteering has continued to this day. The Constitution was suspended during WWII and The Bill of Rights has been suspended also. The Patriot Act is a carbon copy of the German Constitution of 1940 under Hitler. 155,000 Nazis were moved to America under Project Paperclip. You wonder why we have a problem. Franklin Roosevelt created "The United States, Inc." on March 9th, 1933, registered in France and recorded under the Vatican Corporation of Rome. All our alphabet soup agencies are incorporated under the United Nations. They don't work for you. The Shadow Government is always operating with slight of hand and the public is asleep. The big corporations spend billions to get what they want, and the public be damned. It would appear many Congressmen and Senators get their cut of the profits of this organized crime and Big Pharma. And it is said our representatives are preselected and have sworn an oath to the New World Order. I hope that isn't true! Combine corruption with the creeping socialism and Communist conspirators the shelf life of the republic is nearly expired. Our judges are wearing the black robes of their Satanic masters. There is no justice. The situation in Washington, D.C. reads like Dan Brown's novel The Lost Symbol. We are currently engaged in the End Times battle of good and evil prophesied in the Book of Revelations. Now is the time to reestablish freedom and liberty or they will be gone forever. Abraham Lincoln said that "America will never be destroyed from the outside. If we falter and lose our freedoms, it was because we destroyed ourselves."

George Washington also had some words to say about freedom. Washington said, "A free people ought not only be armed and disciplined, but they should have sufficient arms and ammunition to maintain a status of independence from any who might attempt to abuse them which would include their own government." As the Japanese generals believed in WWII that if Americans have a gun behind every blade of grass, then we cannot be conquered. Countries that demand self-defense and freedom like Switzerland, demand every citizen has arms and ammunition to defend the country from invasion.

The Qudos Bank Arena and Olympic Park in Sydney, Australia is host to a mass vaccination of 24,000 12-year-old children. The arena has also been hosting numerous Satanic rock bands and Satanic ceremonies. We believe the mass vaccination (without parents present) is a Satanic ceremony. But Australians have turned in all their guns and are at the mercy of the authorities who wish to sacrifice their children. **DON'T BE LIKE AUSTRALIA!**

I AM NOT ADVOCATING CIVIL WAR OR REVOLUTION. I am advocating preparedness and self-defense. Brue Lee said it best. A student once asked Bruce Lee "You teach me fighting, but you talk about peace. How do you reconcile the two? Bruce Lee beautifully replied "It is better to be a warrior in a garden than to be a gardener in a war."

Therefore, I will leave you here with just one word. **RESIST.** Resist with every fiber of your being. Draw a line in the sand and do not give an inch. You will have to fight for every liberty you give up and it is better not to pay for the same real estate twice. Be a sovereign individual. Support the Constitution with your last breath as it the only protection you have. Defund the United Nations, The CDC, and the World Health Organization, NOT THE POLICE. Never forget we were rebels forged in the battle against tyranny. Vote out anyone who supports lockdowns, masks, vaccines, health IDs, RELOCATION BY TROOPS or home testing. Expose the fraud. Dig deeper into the lives of those orchestrating the fraud. You will be shocked by their connections to Satanism and white slavery. Do your research. I recommend Dr. Richard Flemings book **Is Covid-19 a Bioweapon? A Scientific and Forensic Investigation**. (It is scheduled for release on Sept 7th, 2021. A podcast is available at www.brighteon.com with Mike Adams.) Buy it and follow the trail. Expose them! Boycott any company, airline or cruise ship that supports Health Passports. Serve anyone blocking your travel with Writs of Travel and demand your common law rights. (Available at www. toolsforfreedom.com Order #3381.) Have any official asking questions about you trespassed and jailed.

Any public official that doesn't support your rights guaranteed by the Bill of Rights needs to be charged with treason. Be meticulous in recording public statements that are pro-vaccination for possible Nuremberg style trials in the future for crimes against humanity. Establish 2nd Amendment Sanctuary cities. Form healing groups, study groups, buyers groups and keep informed daily. Mine gold and demand the mint turns it into coin as outlined by our founding fathers in the Constitution. Keep capitalism alive as it works. Be a majority of one. Unplug yourselves from the lies and fake news. Get a second passport. Be a perpetual traveler if you can. Move your assets offshore to the Turks and Caicos Islands. Live off the grid if you can and grow your own food. 12 acres, a horse and a rifle are your best bet for survival when we're thrown back into the 18th century with the next depression.

President Trump was quoted at a recent rally (August 21st.) that "This is a sick culture, and our country is a disaster and its going to die before your very eyes if this craziness isn't stopped in so many ways".

Evil rules the world now, but once thousands of enlightened masters are trained the pendulum will swing back to righteousness and we will defeat them! **Throw a wrench into the hopes of the wicked by being healthy and connected to God.**

The battle sir is not to the strong alone; it is to the vigilant, the active, the brave.

PATRIC HENRY

APPENDIX A:

YOUR POWER TO TRESPASS

BY KRISANNE HALL, JD

IF A GOVERNMENT AGENT OR assignee comes to your property, it will be important to those who wish to protect their privacy and property to **KNOW THEIR RIGHTS**.

- You do not have to answer ANY QUESTIONS or make ANY STATEMENT to ANY GOVERNMENT AGENT or assignee. (5th Amendment of the US Constitution and corresponding section of your State Constitution.)

- Simply asking an agent to identify themselves does not waive your Rights.

- You have the Right to be free from any government agent or assignee entering your property, your home, or your business without a properly obtained warrant. (4th and 5th Amendments of the US Constitution and corresponding sections of your State Constitution.)

- Simply demanding a copy of that warrant does not waive your Rights.

- You have the Right to tell any government agent or assignee to leave your property if they cannot produce a properly obtained warrant. (4th and 5th Amendments of the US Constitution and corresponding sections of your State Constitution.)

- Simply demanding an agent or assignee of the government to leave your property does not waive your Rights.

- If a government agent or assignee refuses to leave your property or returns to your property after being warned against entering or returning, that agent or assignee has committed the crime of Trespass and is subject to arrest. (State Law, 4th & 5th Amendments to the US Constitution and corresponding sections of State Constitution as confirmed by Supreme Court Opinions).

- You have the Right to record through audio, video, or photographic recording of any government agent or assignee on your property, either with or without consent of that agent or assignee. (Multiple Federal Court Opinions recognize that the First Amendment plainly protects the filming of officers and public agents.)

- Please find attached a TRESSPASS WARNING form that you may issue to any government agent or assignee that fails to satisfy the requirement of the US and State Constitutions. HAND THE COMPLETED FORM DIRECTLY TO THE AGENT OR ASSIGNEE WHILE TELLING THEM THEY MUST NOW LEAVE THE PROPERTY AND YOU WILL NOT BE ANSWERING ANY QUESTIONS.

- You should have your address pre-written on the form and as the need arises, fill in the date and time. It is highly recommended that you take a picture of the agent you are serving the warning so you may then prove that this person has been issued a formal Trespass Warning.

APPENDIX B:

TRESPASS WARNING

YOU ARE BEING ISSUED A TRESSPASS WARNING, ANY FUTTHER ENTRY OF THIS PROPERTY WILL BE SUBJECT TO ARREST.

Address of Property: _____

Date and Time of Trespass: _____

Owner/lessee of Property: _____

I have taken a photograph of you to show to a Deputy or Peace Office to prove delivery of this Notice of Trespass.

NOTICE TO THE TRESPASSER

Trespass is a general intent crime that usually required no evidence that the defendant intended to commit the offense. The mere act of willfully entering upon, remaining in, or returning to any property, or after being warned not to do so, is sufficient to establish guilt.

By State law it is a crime if the offender defies an order to leave: if the offender opens a door, fence, or gate.

Notice against trespassers may be provided by posting, fencing, cultivation, or actual communication (warning). See State Laws for the definitions of posting, fencing, cultivation, etc.

Warning may be given by the property owner or by a person authorized to do so by the property owner.

A warning may be in writing or may be verbal. A verbal warning by the property owner or his or her agent is sufficient to constitute warning against remaining in or reentry onto the property.

The inability to issue a written Trespass Warning to the subject does not prohibit a subsequent arrest for trespass if there is evidence through a sworn statement or other evidence to establish when the trespass warning was given and that it was given to the same subject. I have taken a picture of you, to establish evidence of my warning against returning to this property.

By State Law, an officer finding that a previously warned subject has returned to the same property without an invitation to do so may arrest the subject for trespassing.

When a subject has been duly warned to leave or stay off the premises, even if those premises are a BUSINESS ESTABLISHMENT, by law it is safe to assume that any invitation to enter was withdrawn. Any return by the subject, along with a complaint and proof of warning by the owner or agent, justifies a charge of Trespass.

THERE IS NO PERMITTED "FIRST AMENDMENT ACTIVITY" ON PRIVATE PROPERTY OF ANY SORT.

EVEN PERSONS ACTING AS AGENTS OF THE GOVERNMENT MAY BE TRESPASSED.

State and US Constitutions guarantee that every person is to be secure in their property from searches and seizures without a warrant based upon probably cause issued pursuant to the rules of due process. Agents of the government cannot simply enter private property based upon the color of law or a perceived need. The US Supreme Court, June 23, 2021, in **CEDAR POINT NURSERY ET ALL v. HASSID ET AL.** established that a law that allows agents of the government or even permits private citizens the authority to enter property without a warrant or invitation can amount to the taking of that property and is therefore contrary to the Constitution.

YOU HAVE BEEN DULY NOTIFIED- IF YOU RETURN TO THIS PROPERTY YOU WILL BE SUBJECT TO ARREST.

Liberty First Legal, Inc. 7/7/2021. hhps://libertyfirst.legal/

APPENDIX C:

VACCINE MANDATE REFUSAL FORMS

NOTE TO EMPLOYER: As your employee, I am requesting that you review this document, provide the requisite information, and sign the form, in regard to your requirement that employees get a Covid-19 emergency use authorization (EUA) investigational vaccine.

1. If I agree to receive an EUA Covid-19 injection, does my employee **health insurance plan** provide complete coverage should I experience an adverse event, or even death?

   _____

   _____

   _____

2. As an employee, does my **life insurance policy** provide any coverage in the event that I die from receiving an EUA Covid-19 injection?

   _____

   _____

   _____

3. As an employee, will you be providing **Workers' Compensation, disability insurance, or other resources** if I have an adverse event to an EUA Covid-19 injection and am unable to come to work for days, weeks, or months, or if I am disabled for life?

_____

_____

_____

_____

4. **The Food and Drug Administration (FDA) required that EUA vaccine recipients be provided with certain vaccine-specific information to help them make an informed decision about vaccination.** The EUA fact sheets that must be provided are specific to each authorized Covid-19 injection and are developed by the manufacturers of the injections. (Pfizer/BioNTech, Moderna, Oxford/AstraZeneca and the Johnson & Johnson subsidiary Janssen). The fact sheets must provide the most current and up-to-date information on the injections, and vaccine recipients must also receive information about adverse events. Have you read, understood, and provided me (and all other employees" with these fact sheets and with current information on adverse events so that I/we can make an educated decision?

5. **Have you reviewed the available databases of material adverse events reported to date for people who have received Covid-19 injections?** Potential and reported adverse events include death, anaphylaxis, neurological disorder, autoimmune disorders, other long-term chronic diseases, blindness and deafness, infertility, fetal damage, miscarriage, and stillbirth.

_____

_____

_____

_____

6. The FDS's guidance on emergency use authorization of medical products requires the FDA to "ensure that recipients are informed

to the extent practicable given the applicable circumstances. **(t)**
hat they have the option to accept or refuse the EUA prod-
uct...." Are you aware of this statement? Have you informed all
employees that they have the option to refuse?

_____

_____

_____

_____

_____

7. With respect to the emergency use of an unapproved product, the
   Federal Food, Drug and Cosmetic Act, Title 21 U.S.C 360bbb-3
   (E) (1)(A) (ii) (I-III) reiterates that **individuals be informed of**
   the option to accept or refuse administration of the product,
   (and) of the consequences, if any, of refusing administration of
   the product, and of the alternative to the product that are available and of their benefits and risks." If EUA Covid-19 investigation vaccines are ever approved by the FDA, state legislation
   would be required to allow companies to mandate the Covid-19
   injections. Are you aware of these facts?

_____

_____

_____

_____

8. EUA products are unapproved, unlicensed, and experimental. Under the Nuremberg Code- the foundation of ethical
   medicine- no one may be coerced to participate in a medical
   experiment. The individual's consent is absolutely essential.
   No court has ever upheld a mandate for an EUA vaccine. **In**
   Doe #1 v. Rumsfeld, 297 F. Supp. Wd 119 (2003) , a federal

court held that the U.S. military could not mandate EUA vaccines for soldiers." (t)he United States cannot demand that members of the armed forces also serve as guinea pigs for experimental drugs." (Id at 135) Are you aware of this?

---

9. The United States Code of Federal Regulations and the FDA require the informed consent of human subjects for medical research. The EUA Covid-19 injections are unapproved, unlicensed, investigational vaccines that are still in their experimental stage. It is unlawful to conduct medical research on a human being, even in the event of an emergency, unless steps are taken to secure the **informed consent** of all participants. Are you aware of this?

---

10. According to Federal Trade Commission (FTC) Guidelines and the FTC's "Truth in Advertising," promotional material—especially material involving health related products cannot mislead consumers, omit important information, or express claims. All of this falls under the rubric of "deceptive advertising" (whereby a company is providing or **endorsing a product**), whether presented in the form of an ad, or a website, through email, on a poster, or in the mail. For example, statement such as "all employees are required to the Covid-19 vaccine to make the workspace safe" or "it's safe and effective" leave out critical information. Critical information includes the facts that Covid-19 injections are unapproved EUA vaccines that "may" or Many not" prevent Covid, won't necessarily make the workspace safer, and could in fact cause harm. Not providing links or attachment of the

manufacturers' fact sheet and current information on adverse events is omitting safety information. Are you aware of this?

_____

_____

_____

_____

11. Since the Covid lockdowns began over one year ago, there have been over 178 reported breaches of unsecured protected health information (PHI), incidents investigated by the Office for Civil Rights (OCR). These breaches exposed millions of people's personal health information. Although many of these incidents were attributed to hacking, some of the breaches to PHI fell directly under the 1996 Health Insurance Portability and Accountability Act (HIPAA), such as sharing a patient's or person's information with an unauthorized individual or incorrectly handling PHI. **Can you please explain your obligations to me, under HIPAA law, and how you are going to protect my personal information, both with respect to your requirement that I receive this injection?**

_____

_____

_____

_____

12. Whereas pharmaceutical companies that manufacture EUA vaccines have been protected from liability related to injuries or deaths caused by experimental agents since the PREP Act was enacted in 2005, **Companies and all other institutions or individuals who mandate experimental vaccines on any human**

being are not protected from liability. Are you aware that you do not enjoy such liability protection?

_____

_____

_____

_____

_____

13. **Are you aware that employees could file a civil suit against you should they suffer an adverse event, death, or termination from their place of employment?**

_____

_____

_____

_____

14. As the legally authorized officer of the employer/company, I have read all the above information, have provided my employees with all of the information that the FDA requires be provided to recipients of the Covid-19 injections, and **do hereby agree to assume 100% financial responsibility for covering any and all expenses from adverse events, including death, through insurance coverage or directly. In addition, I affirm that the employee with no be subjected to loss of their job should they decline to receive a Covid-19 injection.**

_____

Authorized officer of company requiring injection

_____

_____

Company

_____

Date

_____

Employee

_____

Company

_____

Date

_____

Witness

_____

_____

Company

_____

_____

Date

_____

NOTE: RELIGIOUS EXEMPTION FORMS CAN BE OBTAINED FROM LIBERTY COUNSEL: https://lc.org/exempt and click on "Employment Sample." Or see the October 4th, 2021, issue of The New American pages 16 and 17 published by The John Birch Society to purchase a reprint.

BIBLIOGRAPHY

FOOTNOTES:

(1) Rashid A. Buttar, Dr. The 9 Steps to Keep the Doctor Away: Simple Actions to Shift Your Body and Mind to Optimum Health for Greater Longevity. (GMEC Publishing LLC: Lake Tahoe, Ca. 2010.)

(2) Anonymous. Handbook for the New Paradigm. (Carson City, NV: Bridger House Publishing, undated.)

(3) Frank Arjava Pettter. Reiki Fire: New Information about the Origins of the Reiki Power A Complete Manual. (Twin Lakes, WI: Lotus light/Shangri-La. 1997.) page 113.

(4) Lawrence Frego, Lt. USN. (ret.) An End to All Disease & The DaVinci Code Revelations. (Bloomington, IN: AuthorHouse Publishing 2009) pages 76 & 77.

(5) Wills, Gary. John Wayne's America. (New York, NY) Touchstone. 1998. Page 320.

SUGGESTED VIDEOS FROM WWW.TOOLSFORFREEDOM.COM

3897. FORMER FEMA AGENT REVEALS WHAT COULD BE IN THE COVID VACCINE DVD. $20.00

#3814 LEARN WHY "COVID" IS ATUALLY TOXICITY FROM VACCINES AND EMF EXPOSURE. DVD. $20.00

3592 THE 5G WAR AGAINS HUMANITY DVD. $16.00

#3766 THE Coronavirus PLANDEMIC EXPOSED DVD. $15.00

#3908 HOW THE COVID AGENDA IS ENACTING THE 10 STAGES OF GENOCIDE. DVD. $16.00

#3736 5g Frequencies Affect Your Oxygen Levels, Leading to Same Symptoms as Coronavirus. DVD. $16.00.

And don't forget to order your copy of The Essential Underground DVD directory of over 2,000 Controversial Titles from www. toolsforfreedom.com. $12.95 plus $6.50 shipping and handling from ISA 4-831 Kuhio Hwy. #438-333. Kapaa, Hawaii 96746. (800) 770-8802.

You may also like Ormus Super-greens ½ lb box $39.95. Order # 1035.

Also see report **# 9007 Former Judge Reveals Secrets of America**. $20.00. This is one of the most damning exposes of America ever published.

SUGGESTED WEBSITES:

www.brighteon.com for daily podcasts and updates on Covid-19 by Mike Adams-the Health Ranger. See Dr. Flemings new video about Covid-19 vaccines as a bioweapon.

www.mercola.com Dr. Joseph Mercola

www.americasfrontlinedoctors.com The latest vaccine information and HCQ prescriptions online. Google may redirect your search and lead to prejudiced information about Dr. Simone Gold. Do read her book and get the whole story from her point of view. She is being marginalized as a "notorious antivaxxer" and was arrested for attending the protest at the capitol.

https://home.nra.org. The National Rifle Association.

https://jbs.org. The John Birch Society publishes The New American Magazine and has monthly political updates, particularly on Covid-19.

https://jpfo.org. Jews for the Preservation of the Second Amendment.

https://www.saf.org The Second Amendment Foundation.

www.adventuresunlimitedpress.com Adventures Unlimited Press.

SUGGESTED READING:

Adamo, Christopher. 2019. Rules for Defeating Radicals: Countering the Alinsky Strategy in Politics and Culture. Columbia, SC. Made in the USA.

Adams, Sam. 2008. Understanding and Surviving Martial Law: How to Survive and Even Prosper During the Coming Police State. Collinsville, MS. Heritage Press Publications LLC

Alinsky, Saul D. 1971. Rules for Radicals: A Pragmatic Primer for Realistic Radicals. New York, NY. Vintage Books A Division of Random House.

Anonymous. Undated. HANDBOOK FOR THE NEW PARADIGM. Carson City, NV. Bridger House Publishing.

Anonymous. 2020. Pandemics: A Brief History. Columbia, SC. University Press.

Auman, Catherine. 2017 & 2020. Tantric Dating: Bring Love and Awareness to the Dating Process. Los Angeles, Ca. Green Tara Press.

Baldwin, Ann. 2020. Reiki in Clinical Practice: A Science-based Guide. Pencaitland, Scotland. Handspring Publishing.

Blaisdell, Bob. 2003. The Communist Manifesto and Other Revolutionary Writings: Marx, Marat, Paine, Mao, Gandhi, and Others. Mineola, New York. Dover Publications, Inc.

Bowles, Jeff T. 2021. The Miraculous Cure for and Prevention of All Diseases: What Doctors Never Learned. Unknown. University Science Press.

Bracken, Len. 2002. The Shadow Government: 9-11 and State Terror. Kempton, Illinois. Adventures Unlimited Press.

Brennan, Barbara Ann. 1987. Hands of Light: A Guide to Healing Through the Human Energy Field. New York, NY: Bantam Books.

Brown, Sylvia. 2009. End of Days: Predictions and Prophecies About the End of the World. New York, NY. New American Library/Penguin Group.

Butler, Smedley D. Brigadier General. 1935, 2003. War is a Racket. Port Townsend, WA. Feral House.

Buttar, Dr. Rashid A. 2010. 9 Steps to Keep the Doctor Away: Simple Actions to Shift Your Body and Mind to Optimum Health for Greater Longevity. Lake Tahoe, NV. GMEC Publishing, LLC.

Campobasso, Craig. 2021. The Extraterrestrial Species Almanac: The Ultimate Guide to Greys, Reptilians, Hybrids, and Nordics. Newburyport, MA. Weiser Books.

Carmack, Patrick S. J. 1998. The Money Masters: How International Bankers Gained Control of America. Joplin, MO. Royalty Production Co. (This book is a transcript of the video of the same name.)

Carter, Albert E. 1995. The Miracles of Minerals: The Human Need For Ninety Plus Elements From A Cell's Point of View. Provo, Utah. AIR Publishers.

Childress, David. 2020. Antarctica and the Secret Space Program: From WWII to the Current Space Race. Kempton, Illinois. Adventures Unlimited Press.

Childress, David. 2013. Vimana: Flying Machines of the Ancients. Kempton, Ill. Adventures Unlimited Press.

Coleman, Vernon. 2014. Anyone Who Tells You Vaccines Are Safe and Effective is Lying. Columbia, SC. Made in the USA.

Cooper, Milton William. 1991, 2020. Behold a Pale Horse. Flagstaff, AZ. Light Technology Publishing.

Cori, Patricia. 2001,2008. Atlantis Rising: The Struggle of Darkness and Light. Berkeley, CA. North Atlantic Books.

Cori, Patricia. 2000, 2008. The Cosmos of the Soul: A Wake-up Call for Humanity. Berkeley, CA. North Atlantic Books.

Cori, Patricia. 2017. The New Sirian Revelations: Galactic Prophecies for the Ascending Human Collective. Berkeley, Ca. North Atlantic Books.

Cousins, Gabriel, M.D. 1986. Spiritual Nutrition and the Rainbow Diet. Boulder, CO. Cassandra Press.

Crandall, Chauncey. 2020 Fight Back: Beat the Coronavirus. West Palm Beach, Fl. Humanix Books.

Caumo, Andrew. 2020. American Crisis: Leadership Lessons from the Covid-19 Pandemic. New York, NY. Crown.

Dale, Judge. Undated. Former Judge Reveals Secrets of American: Where Commerce and Justice Collide. Unknown location. Published by The Anti-Corruption Society. #9007 from www.toolsforfreedom. com $20.00

David, John. 2015. Blueprints for Awakening Vol 2: Rare Dialogues with 7 Indian Masters on the Teachings of Sri Ramana Maharshi. London, UK. Open Sky Press.

Davidson, James Dale & Rees-Moog, Lord William. 1997. The Sovereign Individual: How to Survive and Thrive During the Collapse of the Welfare State. New York, NY. Simon & Schuster.

Diamond, Blu. 2021. The Great Reset Hidden Agenda. Philo, Ohio. Universal Mizfits Publishing Inc.

Diamond, Jared. 1997. Guns, Germs, and Steel: The Fates of Human Societies. New York, NY. W.W. Norton & Company.

Diodge, Norman. 2007. The Brain That Changes Itself: Stories of Personal Triumph from the Frontiers of Brain Science. New York, NY. Penguin Books.

Farrell, Joseph P. 2016. Hidden Finance, Rogue Networks and Secret Sorcery: The Fascist International, 9/11, and Penetrated Operations. Kempton, Ill. Adventures Unlimited Press.

Feuer, Elaine. 1996. Innocent Casualties: The FDA's War Against Humanity. Pittsburg, Pa. Dorrance Publishing Co., Inc.

Flanigan, Patrick & Flanagan, Gael Crystal. Undated. Elixir of the Ageless: You are What You Drink. Flagstaff, AZ. Vortex Press.

Foner, Eric. 1995. Paine: Collected Writings. New York, NY. Penguin Random House.

Franklin, Ben. 1758, 1986. The Way To Wealth. Bedford, MA. Applewood Books.

Freeland, Elana. 2018. Under An Ionized Sky: From Chemtrails to Space Fence Lockdown. Port Townsend, WA. Feral House

Frego, Lawrence LT. USN. 2009. An End to All Disease & The DaVinci Code Revelations. Bloomington, IN. Authorhouse.

Fry, T.C. 1989. The Great AIDS Hoax. Manchaca, TX. Health Excellence Systems.

Garrett, Gregory Lessing. 2020. The Age of Deception. Hollister, Ca. Gregory Lessing Garrett Publishing Inc.

Garrett, Gregory Lessing. 2020 The Invisible Enemy. Hollister, Ca. Gregory Lessing Garrett Publishing Inc.

Garrett, Gregory Lessing. 2020. Stand or Fall in the Pandemic Chess Game. Hollister, Ca. Gregory Lessing Garrett Publishing Inc.

Gold, Simone M.D, J.D. & America's Frontline Doctors. 2020. I Do Not Consent: My Fight Against Medical Cancel Culture. New York, NY. Post Hill Press.

Hays, J. Mich'el Thomas. 2013. Rise of the New World Order: The Culling of Man. Samaritan Sentinel Publishing.

Hays, J. Mich'el Thomas. 2015. Rise of the New World Order 2: The Awakening. Samaritan Sentinel Publishing.

Hirschhorn, Joel S. 2021 Pandemic Blunder: Fauci and Public Health Blocked Early Home Covid Treatment. USA. Outskirts Press.

Hogan, Douglas L. 2021. Oath Takers: Book 1 of the Patriot Series. Columbia, SC. Made in the USA.

Hogan, Douglas L. 2021. Surviving Martial Law: Book 2 in the Patriot Series. Columbia, SC. Made in the USA.

Horowitz, David. 2017. Big Agenda: President Trump's Plan to Save America. West Palm Beach, FL: Humanix Books.

Horowitz, Mitch. 2018. The Miracle Club: How Thoughts Become Reality. Rochester, VT. Inner Traditions.

Honervogt, Tanmaya. 1998, 2014. The Power of Reiki: An Ancient Hands-On Healing Technique. New York, NY. St. Martin's Griffith.

Huey, Craig A. 2018, The Deep State: 15 Surprising Dangers You Should Know. Terrance, Ca. Media Specialists.

Hume, 1923, 2017. Ethel D. Bechamp or Pasteur? A Lost Chapter in the History of Biology. Columbia, SC. Made in the USA.

Icke, David. 2017. Everything You Need to Know But Have Never Been Told. Derby, UK. Ickonic Enterprises Ltd.

Kasten, Len. 2017. Alien World Order: The Reptilian Plan to Divide and Conquer the Human Race. Rochester, Vt. Bear and Co.

Keene, Grace J. JD. 2021. The Baha I Faith and Aliens: The Evidence Revealed. Coppell, Tx. Made in the USA.

Kengor, Paul. 2020. The Devil and Karl Marx. Gastonia, NC. Tan Books.

Klinger-Omenka, Ursula. 2010. Reiki With Gemstones: Activating your Self-Healing Powers Connecting the Universal Life Force Energy with Gemstone Therapy. Twin Lakes, WI. Lotus Light.

Koire, Rosa. Behind the Green Mask: U.N. Agenda 21. Santa Rosa, Ca. The Post Sustainability Institute Press.

Korsgaard, Soren Roest. 2020. The Most Dangerous Book Ever Published- Deadly Deception Exposed! Germany. KP Koresgaard Publishing.

Kropotkin, Peter. Undated. The Conquest of Bread. Columbia, SC. Made in the USA.

Lad, Vasant. 1998. The Complete Book of Ayurvedic Home Remedies: Based on the Timeless Wisdom of India's 5,000-Year-Old Medical System. New York, NY. Harmony Books.

Lama, Dalai & Tutu, Desmond. 2016. The Book of Joy: Lasting Happiness in a Changing World. New York, NY. Penguin Random House LLC

Lawlor, Paula. 2010. A Love Devout; The True Untold Story of Mary Magdalene. Del Mar, CA. Magdalene Publishing.

Levin, Mark R. 2021. American Marxism. New York, NY. Threshold Imprints, a division of Simon and Schuster Inc.

Lubeck, Walter. 1997. Rainbow Reiki: Expanding the Reiki System with Powerful Spiritual Abilities. Twin Lakes, WI: Lotus Light/Shangri-La.

Marrone, Paolo. 2016. Ancient Wisdom: The Monk with No Past 2nd Edition. Independently published from the original Italian.

Mars, Jim. 2008. The Rise of the Fourth Reich: The Secret Societies That Threaten To Take Over America. New York, NY. Harper Collins.

Mars, Jim. 2013. Our Occulted History: Do The Global Elite Conceal Ancient Aliens? New York, NY. Harper Collins.

Mars, Jim. 2015. Population Control: How Corporate Owners Are Killing Us. New York, NY. Harper Collins.

Mars, Jim. 2000. Rule by Secrecy. New York, NY. Harper Collins.

Mars, Jim. 2010. The Trillion Dollar Conspiracy: How The New World Order, Man-made Diseases, And Zombie Banks Are Destroying America. New York, NY. Harper Collins.

Mercola, Dr. Joseph. 2020. EMF*D: 5G, Wi-Fi & Cell Phones: Hidden Harms and How to Protect Yourself. Carlsbad, Ca. Hay House.

Mercola, Dr. Joseph. 2021. The Truth About Covid 19- Exposing the Great Reset, Lockdowns, Vaccine Passports, and the New Normal.

Why We Must Unite in a Global Movement for Health and Freedom. White River Junction, VT. Chelsea Green Publishing.

Meyer, Marvin. 2004. The Gospels of Mary: The Secret Tradition Of Mary Magdalene The Companion of Jesus. New York, NY, Harper Collins Publishers.

Miller, Dean. 2017. Deep State: The Truth About the Secret US "Shadow Government" Ruling America And How You Can Fight And Beat It Before They Take Everything From You. Estes Park, CO. 5280 Publishing LLC dba AmericanSurvivor.com.

Mitchell, Krista. 2018. Crystal Reiki: A Handbook for Healing Mind, Body, And Soul. New York, NY. Sterling Publishing Co. Inc.

Mr. X, 2020. Sleeper Cell Secrets of Spies and Our Founding Fathers. Cedar City, UT. Spy Briefing LLC.

Murray, Steve. 2003. Reiki the Ultimate Guide. Las Vegas, NV. Body & Mind Productions.

Ortleb, Charles. Fauci: 2019. The Bernie Madoff of Science and the HIV Ponzi Scheme that Concealed the Chronic Fatigue Syndrome Epidemic. Salem, Mass. Rubicon Publishing.

Orwell, George. 1949 & 1977. 1984. New York, NY. Signet Classics.

Parsa, Cyrus A. The Great Reset: How Big Tech Elites And The World's People Can Be Enslaved By China CCP or A.I. La Jola, Ca. The AI Organization.

Patrick, Sean. 2013. Awakening Your Inner Genius. Columbia, SC. Oculus Publishers.

Patrick, Sean. 2012. The Know Your Bill of Rights Book: Don't Lose Your Constitutional Right. Learn Them! Columbia, SC. Oculus Press.

Perloff, James. 2013. Truth is a Lonely Warrior: Unmasking The Forces Behind Global Destruction. Burlington, Mass. Refuge Books.

Petter, Frank Arjava. 1997. Reiki Fire: New Information about the Origins of the Reiki Power. A Complete Manuel. Twin Lakes, WI. Lotus Light/Shanri-La.

Plumb, Laura 2018. Ayurveda Cooking for Beginners: An Ayurvedic Cookbook to Balance and Heal. Emeryville, Ca. Rockridge Press.

Popper, Pamela A. & Prier, Shane D. 2020. Covid Operation: What Happened, Why it happened, and What's Next. USA. IGCtesting.com.

Quinlan, Heather E. 2020. Plagues, Pandemics, and Viruses: From the Plague of Athens to Covid-19. Canton, MI. Visible Ink Press.

Radin, Dean. 2013 Supernormal: Science, Yoga, and the Evidence for Extraordinary Psychic Abilities. New York, NY. Deepak Chopra Books.

Rama, Swami. 2001. Living with the Himalayan Masters. Honesdale, PA. The Himalayan Institute Pres.

Ray, Sondra & Ray, Marcus. 2016. Babaji: My Miraculous Meetings with a Maha Avatar. Washington, DC & Nashville, TN. Immortal Ray Publications.

Ray, Sondra & Ray, Marcus. 2019. Liberation: Freedom from Your Biggest Block to Pure Joy. Washington, DC & Nashville, TN. Immortal Ray Publications.

Ray, Sondra & Ray, Marcus. 2018. Physical Immortality: How To Overcome Death. Washington, DC & Nashville, TN. Immortal Ray Publications.

Reiss, Dr. Karina & Bhakdi, Dr. Sucharit. 2020. Corona False Alarm? Facts and Figures. White River Junction, Vt. Chelsea Green Publishing.

Richardson, Diana. 2003. The Heart of Tantric Sex. Alresford, Hants, UK. O Books.

Roland, Paul. 2018.The Nazis and the Occult: The Dark Forces Unleashed by the Third Reich. London, UK. Arcturus Publishing Limited.

Schwab, Claus & Malleret, Thierry. 2020. Covid-19 The Great Reset. Geneva Switzerland. Forum Publishing.

Schweizer, Peter. 2018. Secret Empires: How the American Political Class Hides Corruption and Enriches Family and Friends. New York, NY: HarperCollins Publishers.

Siddhanath, Yogiraj Gurunath. 2010. Babaji: The Lightning Standing Still. San Francisco, CA. Siddhanath Forest Ashram.

Siddhanath, Yogiraj Gurunath. 2007. Wings to Freedom: Mystic Revelations from Babaji and the Himalayan Yogis. USA. Alight Publications.

Simpson, James. 2021. Who Was Karl Marx? The Men, the Motives, and the Menace Behind Today's Rampaging American Left. Baltimore, MD. Simpson Publishing.

Skousen, W. Cleon. 1958, 2014. The Naked Communist. Salt Lake City, UT. Izzard Inc.

Slattery, Peter. 2019. Connect to Your Spirit and ET Guides. Columbia, SC. Made in USA.

Snowden, Edward. 2019. Permanent Record. New York, NY. Picador.

Solzhenitsyn, Aleksandr. 1973. The Gulag Archipelago Vol 1. New York, NY. Harper-Perennial Modern Classics.

Stamper, Mel. 2008. Fruit from A Poisonous Tree: Secrets That Were Never To Be Revealed. New York, NY. iUniverse, Inc.

Stein, Diane. 1996. Essential Reiki: A Complete Guide to an Ancient Healing Art. Freedom, CA. The Crossing Press Inc.

Stewart, James B. 2019. Deep State: Trump, the FBI, And The Rule of Law. New York, NY. Penguin Press.

Sutton, Anthony C. 1979. Energy The Created Crisis. USA. Dauphin Publications.

Sutton, Anthony C. 1977. The War on Gold. USA. Dauphin Publications.

Taylor, Ron. 2016. Agenda 21: An Expose Of The United Nations Sustainable Development Initiative And The Forfeiture of American Sovereignty And Liberties. Coppell, Texas. Made in the USA.

Tebb, Scot. 1898. A Century of Vaccination and What It Teaches. London. Swan Sonnenschein & Co. Lim.

Thompson, Arthur R. 2020. China: The Deep State's Trojan Horse in America. Appleton, WI. The John Birch Society.

Thorn, Victor. 2003. The New World Order Exposed. State College, PA: Sisyphus Press.

Toye, Lori Adaile, 2016. The I AM America Atlas: Based On The Maps, Prophecies, And Teachings Of The Ascended Masters. Payson, Arizona, I AM America Publishing and Distributing.

Tzu, Sun. 2006. The Art of War. Columbia, SC. Filiquarian Publishing LLC.

Van Dyke, Lyle Hartford. 1954, 2018. Silent Weapons for Quiet Wars. San Diego, Ca. The Book Tree.

Wilcox, Robert K. 2008. Target Patton: The Plot To Assassinate General George S. Patton. Washington, D.C., Regnery Publishing.

Wills, Garry. 1998. John Wayne's America. New York, NY, Touchstone.

Wood, Patrick M. Technocracy Rising: The Trojan Horse Of Global Transformation. Mesa, AZ. Coherent Publishing LLC.

Yoganada, Paramhansa. 1946/2005. Autobiography Of A Yogi. New York, NY. The Philosophical Library Inc.

Zagami, Leo Lyon. 2016. Confessions of an Illuminati: The Whole Truth About the Illuminati and the New World Order Vol 1. San Francisco, CA. CCC Publishing.

Zagami, Leo Lyon. Undated. Confessions of an Illuminati: The Time of Revelation and Tribulation Leading up to 2020. San Francisco, Ca. CCC Publishing.